The
Power
of
Discomfort

Discover How Greatness Waits on the Other Side of Fear

Manny Languasco

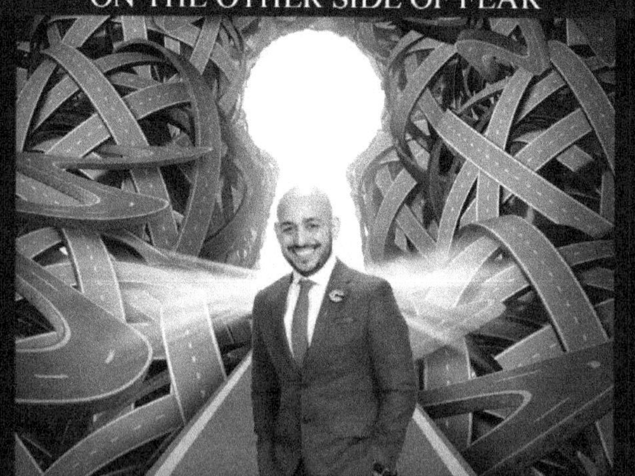

THE
POWER
OF
DISCOMFORT
DISCOVER HOW GREATNESS WAITS
ON THE OTHER SIDE OF FEAR
MANNY LANGUASCO

The Power of Discomfort

ISBN: 9781731289810

CONTENTS

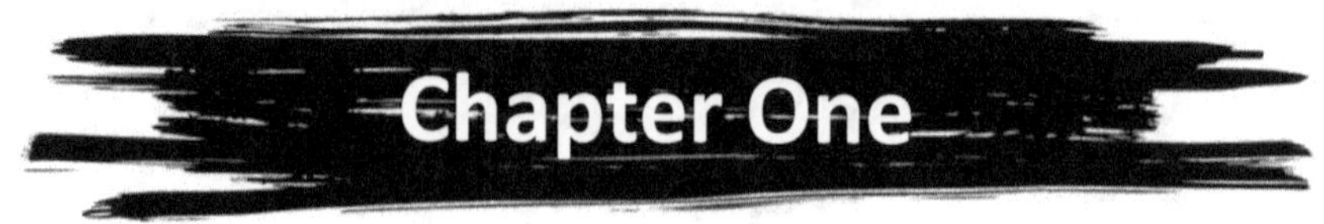

Chapter One

Overcoming Fear

1975

I was born an only child to a poor, uneducated, single mother. My father abandoned us before I was even born. During my first years as a child, we were very poor. As we struggled to find food to eat, my mother not only had to support me but her younger siblings as well. Growing up, I recall seeing my mother beg for money on the streets. She needed a way to feed us. She worked a variety of jobs, always with a smile on her face as if she was not affected by our struggles. Instead, she embraced all challenges without complaints. I cannot imagine how uncomfortable life was for my mother. She was abandoned by both parents at the age of 8 and had to drop out of school to work to support her brothers and sister.

In September 1975, my family lived in Villa Rivas – a typical small town in the Dominican Republic where everyone knew each other. The people counted down the days until Sunday, so they could show off their best clothes at the park and in church. My mother was pregnant with me, expecting a little girl. Even though I turned out to be a boy, she was happy I was healthy, while nervous to have a newborn baby.

She was excited. But she was just 18 years old, without a clue how she'd support her new child. My mother had fallen deeply in love with my father from the very moment she saw him. And as she laid in the hospital bed, enduring the pain of contractions, she couldn't focus, too many things were coming to her mind. She had a sudden flashback and began to recall everything she had gone through as a child.

As the second of six children, she remembered her father coming home drunk, stumbling and hitting her mother in the face. Unsure of what had happened, she'd watch her mother cry inside the closet. This scene would repeat each time her father came home. She vividly remembered the day he packed up his clothes and left the house. At that young age, she began to live an uncomfortable life. When her father left, she thought things would clear up and get better. In her mind, she thought her family would live a better life, so she was thankful. A few months had passed, and her mother met another man. He was tall and handsome, and she was in love. He invited her to move to another city, but he wanted her to leave her kids. Without hesitation, her mother packed her bags and did exactly that. She left her children alone to fend for themselves. All six of them.

Through the pain my mother was experiencing in the hospital, she remembered her two-year-old sister who, at the time, had just began to walk. She remembers seeing her crying and walking behind the car as her mother left, begging her not to leave. Meanwhile, the rest of the siblings were lined up on the side of the street, watching as their mother left them for another man, a stranger. Tears filled her eyes and she fell to the ground. The car disappeared into the distance. She waited for her mother to look back, to stop the car and return. Her mother never turned around or even looked back to see her children one last time. These were the thoughts racing through my mother's mind while she laid in the hospital bed. And there, she promised herself one thing right before I was born: "I will never separate myself from my child until he or she is grown, and I will do whatever it takes to ensure my child does not go through life the same way I did."

When I was growing up, there were many nights I would eat at my friend's house because there was nothing to eat at home. His parents were very kind and treated me as their son. They always had something for me to eat. On several occasions, they helped me with my homework and gave me a place to sleep. I was very close to their entire family, and their kindness influenced me in many ways. Often, I would wear my friends' clothes because I had none at home. Other children would tease me and call me "pio," meaning "rompio" or "broken" because my clothes were tethered and old. This nickname stuck with me until I was a teenager. Very few people knew my real name back then.

As a child, my mother protected me. Even with our lack of money, she tried hard to give me anything I wanted or needed. I always knew and felt how much she loved me. I know she did not want me to go through the hardships she endured as a child. She cared about me, showed love in every single moment of my life, and we were never separated. She never went anywhere without me. She sacrificed herself to the point that she never dated anyone until I was a teenager. My mother dedicated herself to taking care of her family. From a young age, she'd always try and teach me life lessons. She'd say to me: "If you want to be successful in life you have to keep yourself moving. Success is like riding a bicycle, if you do not move you will fail." She influenced my life in so many ways. She made me feel as if we were rich, even though she was struggling to provide shelter and food.

As I got older, I grew curious, like any child. I would often ask her about my grandparents. I wanted to know them. On several occasions, I asked her why my friends have grandparents and I didn't? She always replied with the same answer: "One day, when you are grown up, I will tell you what happened." I was also curious about my father. When I was about 7 years old, I began to wonder why my friends' families had both a mother and a father. I wanted to be like them: I wanted a father to play with, to talk with and to spend time with. I grew frustrated, almost distraught, and begged my mother to tell me where he was.

I was brought up using my mother's last name. I'd write it on tests at school and introduce myself with it. One day at school, I realized my friends would use their fathers' names. Why was I different? Again, my mother said: "One day I will explain it to you." It became a burning desire for me to know, and I kept asking, nagging at her almost every day. I was so persistent that one day she finally broke down and told me that I had a father, and he lived in San Francisco, an adjacent city in the Dominican Republic. That day I was shocked. I thought he was either dead or that she didn't know who my father was, but at last, the truth. He only lived an hour away from my rural town. I immediately told mom : "I want to see him." I wanted to know my father, to have him be a father. She said: "I do not know if he will be able to meet us. He has an important job and is a very busy man." I was confused. How could a man knowingly have a child and not want to meet him or spend time with him? It didn't make sense that he knew about me and never came to see me. My mother's excuses didn't make sense either. Every time I insisted on seeing him, she would shut it down. One day, she relented and agreed to take me to meet him.

Looking back now I realize how momentous this was for her. She had to face her fear of approaching a powerful man with the son he had abandoned, that he never wanted to know, but she faced her fear because she loved me, and that taught me an important lesson: Facing our fears is how we overcome any challenge. Not facing your fear will leave you with regrets. Eventually, questions will arise. I think about my life; how different it would have been today if I did not have the courage to step out of my comfort zone. Outside of your comfort zone is where the growth happens. The reality is; in order to make progress in life, we have to embrace discomfort. Every discomfort or pain delivers awareness of life, and an opportunity for growth. Let your discomfort and pain push you into something new. Let your discomfort lead you into new directions. Let it fuel you to achieve greatness.

1982

I remember feeling so excited that; I could not believe that I would be meeting my father for the first time. I was so happy I went to see my best friend, Fernando to share the news. I told him and his family that I had a father, and I would be meeting him the next day. It was like a gift; An answer to my prayers. The day before, I did not know he existed, but now, I was about to meet him for the first time! I went to bed early that night because I wanted the night to pass quickly. I needed to be ready in the morning and be perfect to meet my father. I wanted him to love me the same as my mom loved me and be so proud of the son he had. I thought about what I would say, but most importantly I imagined how happy he would be when he saw me for the first time. I believed that he would hug me, smile and kiss my cheek. I hoped that he would say that he wanted us to live with him, and how much he missed me. This was a magical moment, my perfect scenario.

The morning finally came, and we took the hour-long bus ride to the city. It felt like the longest bus ride of my life. On the way, I asked my mom so many questions about him. What did he look like? How tall was he? Is he nice? Will he love me? I remember my mom being uncomfortable, but I was so young and excited. I did not realize what her discomfort meant. Looking back, I know she was worried about the reception we would receive. This moment was an awkward moment for her. She had not seen him since her pregnancy when he told her that he was getting married to his girlfriend and wanted nothing to do with the child. As you can imagine that moment was devastating for her.

We finally arrived in the city. We exited the bus and walked the rest of the way to his office. My father was the head of the Department of Agriculture, and his office was in a large government building. We walked inside, and my mother approached his secretary explaining she was there to see him with his son. He made us sit and wait for about two hours! I could not imagine what was going through my mother's mind, but I was still so nervous and excited. After a while, my mother started to get upset and lose her patience. I noticed that something was not right. There was a moment when I saw her face; she looked distraught, so I told her that we could leave. She was probably asking herself so many questions.

Finally, the secretary communicated to us that we could go in. We walked into his huge office. I was so impressed! That was the first time I had seen an office in my life. There were beautiful pictures hanging on the walls and a massive oak desk where he handled his important work. I was flabbergasted! I looked around while my mom was apologizing and explaining the reason why we were there. I remember him looking at me, but I was so nervous I did not know what to do. I was looking around avoiding direct eye contact, and at the same time, I was listening to the conversation between my mother and father. I was waiting for him to stand up from his chair to hug me. I froze and kept looking at him while he just kept staring at me. He finally stood up. He reached into his pocket and pulled out 30 pesos. He gave it to my mother and said, "Here is some money in case you need it. Now you can leave because I have much work to do." With an angry look on her face, my mom walked over to his desk and placed the money on it. She looked him in the eyes and said, "My son is already almost seven years old, I have never asked you for any money. What makes you think I am going to ask you now?" She immediately grabbed me by the hand we walked out of his office. As she was pulling me out, I was looking back at him. He never once looked up to see us leave.

What do you do when you have a dream, and everything is not going the way you planned?

On the long bus ride home, my mom cried the entire time. She apologized for giving me a horrible father. I remember the sun was shining and reflecting off the tears on her face. I did not really understand what just happened. I didn't even get a chance speak with my father. Yes, I got to see him, but I was so sad that I had placed my mother in that situation. I kept telling her I was sorry repeatedly. I wanted to make her feel better, and at the same time, I felt as if the world had ended. Facing this challenging moment for us was the beginning of a major change in my life.

"Each of us must confront our own fears; we must come face to face with them. How we handle our fears will determine where we go with the rest of our lives. We will either experience our life's greatest success and accomplishment or we will be limited by the fear of it."

Before that day everything was great. I was a happy child living in a perfect world with minimal problems. However, looking back I am grateful that I went through this situation at a young age. After that day my life changed. I spent much time alone. I was so disappointed with myself, with the father God had given me and the entire situation. I did not want to speak with anyone. I did not want to share with my friends what he had done to us. On that day, I made a promise. I promised God that when I had kids, I would love them more than anything. There were so many things that came to mind. I felt so angry, but I kept it to myself for years. I remember everyday sitting alone in our backyard, looking at the sky, asking God "why me? Why did this have to happen to me? Why was I poor?" Is this the life God had planned for me? I was frustrated with my circumstances. What I did not know was that God was preparing me for what was to come.

That experience left a very negative impact on me. It was the birthplace that housed many of my fears. I didn't speak to my mom for days, and our relationship changed. My grades in school dropped, and I became distracted. I lost much of the joy I had as a child. I started to blame her because he was such a horrible man. Overcoming that pain and anger was a significant challenge for me.

As time passed, our circumstances didn't improve. We lived in a ramshackle wooden house. The roof was so damaged that when it would rain, it rained inside the house too. While he was living in a beautiful house with his other family, we were living a life of hardship and poverty. Even with all the hardship, she never once complained. As I grew older, my fears continued to take root. I started to believe there were limitations to what I could achieve. These fears manifested in my father's rejection. They grew from the actions and opinions of family and friends, from school and the environment I lived in. Soon, I was surrounded and drowning in those fears. What I did not realize at the time was life is an ongoing journey. I was killing my limitless potential because fear of the unknown and lack of belief in myself. This fear has caused me to falter at certain points in my life. I became a shy and fearful child. I didn't participate in school, and I didn't speak in conversations. I became so quiet that people started to think that I was stupid or mentally retarded. I was constantly afraid. I saw limitations in everything and everyone. As children, we are born without fear. We'll try anything and do anything. It's our experiences in life that teach us to be afraid. Life had dealt me a severe blow, which completely changed me from a fun-loving, excited child, to a poor-spirited creature that saw failure in everything. I was unwilling to do or try anything new. You may ask what happens to us? Why are we afraid of change, to try new things, to get out of our comfort zone, to take risk?

She later told me that she realized she had no one to rely on. She had to be both mother and father and was solely responsible for my care. She became a different woman after visiting my father. She was a harder woman since that fateful day even more protective than before. She was very strict and controlled everything around me. Not out of meanness, but because she loved me so fiercely. She wanted to protect me. My father dealt us a painful blow, but her anger and strength made her determined to take care of me. I saw the change in her. When I would make a childish mistake, her reaction would be harsher than it was before.

One day, she sent me to the market to buy three eggs for dinner. I went and bought the eggs, but as a young boy not thinking, I put them in my pocket. My only thought was to get home quickly. I started running, and as you would expect, all three eggs broke. We had very little money, and of the little we had, I had just carelessly wasted it. When I made it home, I walked through the door with wet pockets, and eggs were dripping down my legs. It was a childish mistake, but because of it, we did not have almost nothing to eat for dinner. She was very hard on me that night, and almost every day. She was so upset, she called me stupid. My father's rejection made me feel inadequate. I believed he didn't want me. My mother said it, my teachers said it, and even some of my friends said it. I honestly started to believe that I was stupid myself. It got to the point where my mother gave me medication because she believed I was mentally impaired.

Sometimes her methods were not the best, because she had no example to learn from. However, every action she took was rooted in her deep love for me. Whenever we went somewhere, she would tell me to sit and not move. She wanted me to be respectful and stay out of trouble. One time, I was sitting in a chair at her friend's house and realized that I really needed to go to the bathroom. I was so afraid to move that I ended up wetting my pants. I was too afraid to open my mouth and speak, even to ask permission to go to the bathroom. You can see why people thought I was stupid.

Her strictness and the negative opinions of those around me provided a fertile breeding ground for my fears and insecurities. At this point, everyone thought I was idiotic, and they did not hesitate to call me dumb. My fear caused me to spend so much time alone that I was always dreaming. In my mind, I created the world I wanted to live in. Having so little, my dreams were filled with thoughts of a better life. I would visualize the home I wanted to have, the car I wanted to drive, the clothes I wanted to wear, and the wife and family I would someday have. I didn't want the same life for them that I had, so I dreamed BIG! Like life so notoriously does, it intruded on my dreams, so I still had my fears and insecurities to conquer. One day while sitting at the edge of the river, observing the water and the little fish swimming along with the current, I thought about the direction my life was headed and why. As I looked into the water, I started reflecting on my fears and the things that I was missing out on because of the them.

Take Control and Keep it Moving

At that point, I thought to myself: No matter what my circumstances are right now, if I want to achieve my dreams I have to keep moving. Then I recalled something that my mother had always told me. She always said, "It does not matter what type of person you are now; what matters the most is whom you want to become." Our situations in life do not determine our future. They only stay with us for as long as we allow them to. For that reason, we need to let things go, learn from our mistakes and move forward. The past is the past and nothing we do can change that. We can learn from it and grow. It is an opportunity to learn. You either take action to ensure you don't make the same mistake twice or you sit back and don't do anything about it. Some things in life we have control over, but other things we don't.

 Growing up without a father in a low-income family was out of my control. What I did have control over was what I did with the situation, how I handled it and how I tried to understand the reason behind it. I could either complain about it for the rest of my life and blame everyone else, or I could take responsibility, take action and face the challenges life was placing in front of me. I decided I wasn't going to be another statistic and continue blaming my mother, my father and the fact that I was poor. I had to adapt to a new way of life, not worry about what I did not have control over and accept what I did have control over. On that day, I decided to make a drastic change. I had to stop complaining about everyone, and I had to hold myself accountable. Not blaming others is the first step in overcoming a fear. Complaining doesn't solve any problems. It doesn't allow us to grow and move forward. When we're afraid, we don't allow ourselves to take risks, to try new things, discover new talents and abilities we didn't know we were capable of. Fear is a limitation; it comes from expecting the worst, from our insecurities, past experiences, someone that we know, or something we've heard. You must take on every situation with a positive mindset. I decided that day I would face my fears.

"The way to develop self-confidence is to do the things you fear and get a record of successful experiences behind you. Success is not a matter of chance, it is a matter of choice; it is not something you sit and wait for. It is something you go out and achieve."

Don't Be Afraid to Make Mistakes

First, I forgave myself for any mistakes I had made (or would make in the future). I didn't need to be perfect. "It's better to have tried and failed than never to have tried at all." It's ok to make mistakes, but what's not ok is to make the same mistake twice, you must learn from them. It was not an easy decision to make; it had been difficult to speak in front of the class, and to raise my hand when I had to. Those were uncomfortable moments for me, but I knew when I was not feeling comfortable, that meant I was growing. If I would have chosen to stay comfortable my life would have not been as it is today. Failure teaches us to overcome obstacles and rebuild our mind while growing and improving habits, believes and strategies.

1989

As a teenager, I started to outgrow my childhood programming. I no longer believed in negative opinions others had of me. Even though I was still shy, my dreams formed into determination to grow and become more. Something inside of me had to change to have a future. I knew I would turn the dreams I had conceived into reality. I wanted to show everyone what they thought about me was wrong.

I wanted to prove it to the world, but I didn't know how to start. Above all, I wanted and needed to prove it to myself. I didn't want to raise a family in the same situation that I had been raised in. I wanted to give them a better life, a better environment and show them all the possibility's life had to offer.

Find Your Why

I found the perfect motivation to challenge myself, to get out of my comfort zone and to leave my old life behind for a new life. I was not doing it for myself; I was doing for my children. Sometimes in life, we need to find a reason that gives us the motivation we need to overcome our obstacles. For me, it has always been leaving a legacy for my family. I want my family to be proud of me and the man I have become, despite the negative circumstances I had to endure. What is your motivation? If you don't have one, find it. It could be a new car, a new house, a vacation, expensive clothes, anything. Whatever it is, it should give you a reason to wake up every morning. What I knew was that in order to make my dreams a reality, I would have to face my fears. I would have to make a fundamental change in my actions, my beliefs, and my circumstances. I would have to become the person I dreamt of and envisioned. I would have to be reborn.

When I was around 14 years old, I was reflecting on my life and the changes I needed to make to achieve my goals. I realized I needed to move away from home if I wanted to achieve anything in my life. Living in a small town, I didn't know anyone who could teach me the fundamentals of how to build a successful life, and more importantly, how to face and overcome my fears. I needed a place where no one knew me, and I would be free to become the person I wanted to be.

I loved my mother dearly. She was my hero, and it was a hard decision to make, but as a young man, I was ready for a change. I was about to make the first of many difficult choice in my life. I knew this was going to make me uncomfortable, but if I didn't take this chance, I would never be able to become the person I envisioned myself to be. Although I was scared to approach her, I would have to let her know that her only son, the child that she had been protecting wants to move out of the house at the age of 14. At this point, I didn't know what to do, but one thing I was sure of was that I wanted to discover what the world had to offer me. I sat with her and told her about the move, and my desire to do something different: to travel, to get to know people, the need to make mistakes, to fail, to be my true self. She immediately asked me if I were crazy, because she would never let me make this stupid decision. She asked me, "where are you going to go? How are you going to support yourself? How are you going to survive?" But most importantly, she asked me, "what do I want to do?" Then she brought up the possibility of my dad asking about my whereabouts, and she would not know how to respond.

Honestly, now I had a big problem to face. I needed a solution, but I didn't know anyone that could help me. I was committed to making that change. I knew inside that my life would be different if I moved out. No one would judge me, and if I moved to another city, I could start all over again without prejudices. Every day, I closed my eyes and imagined me 30 years old living with my mother, not making my dreams reality, waiting for her to provide me with food and money. I said no way, not me. At that moment I had an idea. I thought about God, because I had heard that he helps people to find solutions. I thought, I am going to talk to God, he will help me. Why wouldn't he help me? That question stayed in my head. So, I started going to church every day after school to find a solution to my problem. At that point, I didn't have a relationship with God. I never went to church with my mom. My only spiritual exposure was praying with my mom at night before bed, thanking God for what we had and asking Him to provide for us the next day.

When I went to church, I would pray and talk to God, asking Him to help me find a solution for overcoming my fears. Through prayer, I found a friend. He became someone that I could confide in. I was able to share with him my challenges, insecurities, and concerns. He became my best friend, and we developed a close relationship.

After a couple of months of visiting church, I was praying and honestly, I was about to give up on God, but I asked God for his help in changing the direction of my life. I didn't know how to do this; I thought I was doing something wrong and I needed his help. I didn't want to give up, but I thought he was not listening to me, but on that day while I was praying, a fantastic thing happened. As I was kneeling there, lost in my prayers, I felt a tap on my shoulder. A deep voice said, "Son, do you need some help?" I froze. I was so scared that I didn't want to look behind me. Think about a 14-year-old boy sitting by himself in a huge church, speaking with God, asking for an answer. Then, he hears a voice. I was so scared I almost fell on the floor. I stayed still, waited a little longer before turning to look to my side. As I was waiting, so was he, before he repeated his question. My body was shaking. I was sweating and almost peed in my pants. I thought that God was there speaking to me because he had a deep voice. It was a voice I'd never heard before, plus he didn't sound like he was from the same area. I finally gathered my courage and slowly turned around. It was a big man, over six-feet tall, in his early 30s with a long beard, wearing a white Cassock. His name was Marcos and he was a priest.

"Be willing to step outside your comfort zone every now and then; and take the risks in life that seem worth taking. The outcome may not be as predictable if you'd just have planted your feet and stayed, but it will definitely be more rewarding."

Everyone Needs a Mentor

I didn't realize at the time, but on that day, I met my very first mentor. He was the first person in years that didn't make me feel slow. He was new in town and didn't know anything about me, with him, I was able to be myself. For the first time, I was free to leave behind the expectations and preconceived notions of others and express myself as the young man I was. His guidance had a profound effect on my life, especially over the next few years.

In an effort to turn my life around, I became more involved with the church. I often spoke with the Marcos, the priest, who became a father figure to me. We spent a great deal of time together. He taught me the fundamentals of discipline. We'd wake up at 4:30 each morning to run around the town. When he asked me the first time to wake up at 4:30, I thought he was crazy, but I thought if I wanted to change my life, I needed to change my habits.

"Sometimes you have to go through temporary discomfort and make temporary sacrifices; in order to get long term success and comfort. Confront your discomfort and your fear to see and experience your potential. Reach beyond. Don't limit yourself. When we get too comfortable, that's when we stop seeing the possibilities. "

Soon I found out how amazing it was waking up before anyone. While others are sleeping you are doing something productive and getting a head start on life. It felt so good knowing I was doing the right thing. I enjoyed waking up early and going for a run and praying while most of the people were still sleeping. I felt different, and that's what I was searching for. I was craving change and at my young age, he was offering me what I was looking for at that time. We fasted for days at a time. We would visit other Christian churches and he'd stop the car halfway and we'd walk with the rest of the way. A couple of times during the summer with the Dominican Republic heat blazing down on us and the temperature over 100F, he'd turn the heat on in the car instead of the air conditioner to help "build my character." He always said, "If you want to achieve anything important in your life, you must be willing to make a sacrifice. Great things do not come overnight; it takes discipline, consistency, and desire."

At the time, I thought it was a game. It was fun facing all those challenges, but later realized this was practice helping me get out of my comfort zone. He was laying a foundation of knowledge and principles I would use during my life. He prepared me for the future I would be facing. I didn't know it at the time, but I would lean heavily on the lessons he taught me during the hardships I went through when I moved to the United States. In that short period of time, he became the father figure I never had. I spent more time with him than my family. He was my family. He came into my life for a purpose, and he had been a fantastic friend, father, and mentor. I am so thankful to have had him in my life.

Sometimes I think about my life, and I can't figure out how it would've been without him and his positive influence on me. I've been through so many challenges. I've had to face difficulties and I have had to reinvent myself a few times. I know that without the life lessons I received from him, I wouldn't be here teaching you. I would probably be working a minimum-wage job, possibly addicted to drugs, alcohol or who knows. After he came into my life, it started to have meaning, and every day I had something to look forward to. One day I sat with him and shared all my desires and my insecurities. He agreed to help me overcome some of my fears and help find a solution to move out. Honestly, I was having a lot of fun having a "father" for the first time, but I also knew I needed to fulfill my dreams. I still wanted to travel the world and become a person of influence that positively impacted others through mentorship. When you have a major desire, you have to continue trusting that one day it will come to you. You must prepare for this opportunity, because it's better to be ready for an opportunity and not have one than to have an opportunity and not be ready for it.

One day I asked him: "what is good luck?" He replied with an answer that stuck with me. He said: "Think of luck as two roads going next to one another in the same directions, but at some point, both roads get together, that is good luck." At first, I didn't understand, but he also said: "you drive the car of preparation and your destiny will drive the car of opportunity and if your driving is slower than your destiny, the good luck will never come for you." At that point, it became clearer. If I wasn't ready for the opportunity to meet me, I would always watch it pass right by me without a chance to ever succeed my dreams. I knew he was right. I needed to prepare myself, drive as fast as I can to catch up to my destiny or even better, be ready for the day it came looking for me.

He knew I was shy, so he worked to help me face the challenge. He said: "The only way you are going to overcome your fears is if you deal with them." At that age, I didn't understand much, but he gave me an example saying: "If you are afraid of dogs, then you have to go and get two big dogs as pets. The only way that you will overcome your fears is by confronting them." He was very wise. He taught me that we could not expect to be good at something if we did not dare to start working on it consistently, with discipline and sacrifice. This is something he made me practice every day. To help me overcome my shyness, he made me stand up and talk during any celebration or gathering we attended. I would talk about a Psalm or anything relevant to the occasion. After a while, I gained confidence in myself. I saw there was a world full of possibilities for me to experience. Now I saw my dreams being possible; they were in reach.

"One great enemy we must all endeavor to fear not conquering is fear. Fear can cripple our purpose. Fear asks question we must fear. Fear makes vision a nightmare. One must always cross the barrier of fear to get to the great place of true purpose. For a great number of us who are unable to accomplish this, it's because we are unable to cross the barrier of fear in the first place."

Sometimes in life, we have to do what is difficult and what we least expect to achieve our goals. I didn't want to be shy for the rest of my life. I wasn't willing to allow the fact that we were poor, that

I didn't have a father or that people called me dumb, to determine the course of my life. I was willing to work to make my dreams become a reality. His effect on my life was so profound that I decided to join the seminary. I firmly believed at that moment God wanted me to help him in a big way. Going into the seminary was a huge decision and it meant not having the four kids that I had always been dreaming of. That day I rushed to see my mother to give her the good news. I sat with her and said, "Mom I want to become a priest." As I expected, my mother was against it. She wanted a family and grandchildren, but I was determined to fulfill my new dream, and I would not give up. So, I went to the priest and told him my mother said "yes" to me joining, but she needed to speak with him first. It was a small lie, but I knew she couldn't say no to him. With some discussion and compromise, I accomplished my second goal in my life and was admitted into the seminary at the age of fifteen.

Never Give Up

The seminary was the start of my transformation. It was the confirmation of believing anything was possible for me. I was ready to overcome the obstacles within myself and learn the many lessons necessary to lead a successful life. The first few months were difficult for me. I cried myself to sleep every night. I would go to the roof and look at the sky, thinking about my mother, missing her so much. I missed my friends, my mentor and everything I had left behind. I knew leaving home was the right decision for me. It was a difficult challenge. It was an uncomfortable decision to say the least. I'm not going to lie, there were many days I wanted to give up, but instead, I learned from my mother's example. She never gave up on anything, so I wasn't going to give up either. It was a very uncomfortable situation. I attended seminary for four years. I faced many fears, but most importantly, I met several amazing people. It was a great experience sharing the same goals with hundreds of young men my age, all from different backgrounds and cultures. It was not easy at that young age to face my fears but dreams only become a reality when we get out of the comfort zone. In the seminary, I discovered I was a natural leader. During my time there, I led several youth groups, met fantastic teachers that helped me to develop my mind and laid a solid foundation to prepare me for the rest of my life. They taught me discipline and helped me to challenge myself to be better than I was the day before. I cannot imagine my life without the experiences I attained in the seminary. I learned the fundamentals of honesty, hard work, discipline, dedication, determination, decision and desire. These seven steps were the foundation for facing my fears and any obstacles that have occurred in my life.

I enjoyed my time there, but under the pressure and influence of my friends, I did not take my final vows. Leaving the seminary was another difficult decision. I firmly believe I was born to help others, and at the time, I thought that meant becoming a priest. There was one big problem: Yes, I want to help others, but also, I wanted to have a family. I still dreamt of having children and finding the love of my life. So, I left the seminary to attend college in the big city, where I learned a valuable life lesson that changed my life and stuck with me to this day.

"There is no growth without change. You've got to let go of some of the old stuff. Often when you're experiencing the most pain, you realize it's coming from trying to control everything or resisting the changes that come with progress. But then you see that light. That beautiful next level and when that is what you have to focus on, incredible things happen."

1994

I left the seminary at the age of 19 and decided to attend college. My dream at the time was to study law. I was excited and knew this would make my mother proud and most importantly I would be happy. I was convinced this was what I wanted to do the rest of my life. I saw myself becoming a successful lawyer. I had seen other lawyers from low-income families like mine, and they were living a good life. If I saw someone was successful, I automatically thought I wanted to do the same thing. I convinced myself that I loved whatever career created success for them - and could create success for me. I changed the course of my life and replaced my priorities because of this. It happened many times throughout my life. It may have been a result of not having a father to look up to, that could have helped me figure out exactly "who" I was and help me to find myself. What I experienced during this chapter of my life taught me to stop trying to be someone else and start becoming the man I needed to be. Because of the influence of others, I wasted a lot of time, money, and had many setbacks I sometimes wonder where my life would be today if I had made a different choice.

It was a sunny day in September 1994. I remember it as if it were yesterday, riding the bus with my best friend, Fernando. We hopped on the bus, leaving behind the small rural town where we grew up. We had a two-hour ride to the city where I would start the next chapter of my life. We mostly grew up together, spending so much time together that we were as close as brothers. We would sleep over at each other's houses. We always supported each other. We ate together, did homework together, and even shared clothes. He was the kind of friend that if I had money and he did not, I would give him whatever I had. He was like family, the brother I never had. Fernando was two years older than me and because of this he was already in college by the time I decided to attend. He had an apartment in the city close to the college campus, so I arranged to live with him. I was excited to be reunited with him again. Thinking about studying at the same school, living in the same house - it felt like we were kids again. Brothers like before. The only difference was, he studied computer programing, and I would be studying law. We had been separated for the four years I attended seminary, so we were eager to catch up on all the news and happenings in our lives. Since he already had experience, he shared all kinds of advice on how to handle myself once I reached the big city.

Be Confident in Your Decisions

There was one topic that he was very passionate about and spent much time talking on. It caught my attention and fired up my imagination. He spoke about computers and how they would revolutionize the world. He explained that every school, business, household, and government entity would come to rely on computers. Honestly, we are living his vision right now. Computers would change the course of life as we knew it, and if I did not learn how to use one, I would be behind the times and completely outdated. He was so passionate and confident in his knowledge that he excited and inspired me, but he also planted a seed of doubt. I began to ask questions, was I following the right path in studying Law? Am I really meant to become a lawyer? He went on to tell me there were many lawyers, but very few computer programmers and how he was going to be in high demand once he left college. You should have seen him speaking about it with confidence and passion. It inspired me. Remember, as a poor kid coming from a small rural town, I had never even seen a computer, much less touched one. I was excited and fascinated by what he told me, and the more I listened the more miserable I felt. He spoke with such conviction, he shook my confidence in the major I decided to study. I envisioned myself as a poor lawyer with no clients in an empty office, struggling to make money because of all the competition. Then, I visualized him being a successful programmer, making tons of money working for a large corporation and getting everything, he ever wanted in life.

That night I couldn't sleep. I was up all-night thinking about our conversation, imagining myself in an office sitting in front of a computer unable to figure out how it worked, feeling stupid and miserable. I wondered if I was making the right decision to become a lawyer. I ran all the possible scenarios and weighed the pros and cons. It was 5am, and I was still agonizing, with my mind in turmoil. I was restless and got up and went outside into the garden. I did not know what to do. I needed some help in making the right choice. During this period my mentor, Marcos, was not around. He was studying in Brazil, and I had not spoken with him for years. I didn't know who to call to ask for advice to help me to decide about my career and most importantly to clarify my doubts and insecurities. So, I picked a flower and started to pull the petals off one by one to see which curriculum I would be registering for.... Law (pluck), computers (pluck), law (pluck), computers (pluck). After I finished plucking the last petals, I still wasn't sure what to do. I killed that poor flower for nothing. I went back inside, got a cup of coffee and tried to make a final choice.

Later that morning, I went to the college to register what supposed to be the beginning of my future. I waited in line, nervous, sweating because there was no air conditioning. I thought to myself, 24 hours ago I knew what I wanted, but now I was not sure what I wanted to do for the rest of my life! It was now my turn. I filled out the application, writing all my personal information and then I paused. I had to enter my career choice. I sat there for five minutes trying to buy more time. Doubt and indecision ate at me. With sweat running down my face, I could not stand the thought that if I made the wrong decision how my life would be ruined. I finally made my choice. In the end, I chose computer programming.

The following week, I started the journey to my new career convinced that I was going to change the world and that I was doing the right thing. In my mind, I thought I was going to be successful, and I would be running the IT department for a big corporation. However, within a few months I started to feel miserable. I was not learning anything, and little by little I was losing my passion about the college. I was wasting time and money.

As the time passed, I felt worse and worse, but I was stubborn, and I did not want to give up. I did not want to disappoint my mother, but the truth was, that I was so disappointed in myself. I could not believe I made the wrong decision. I kept going trying and trying. I did not want to give up. I wanted to be someone, but in life you must do what you love, and we should not allow others to make the decisions for us. It was a very confusing time for me. I felt restless and I was starting to become distracted. I was searching for a purpose, for something to motivate me to not give up. Honestly, I was looking for an excuse to drop out of college. I did not want to continue wasting my time, energy, and money doing something that I did not like. I lost interest in getting my degree, in becoming successful and changing the world. My disillusionment with school fueled my interest in girls. My priorities changed, in that I spent more time dating girls than I did studying. My life started going in the wrong direction. All my drive and purpose disappeared. Focusing my time and effort on dating girls, a was not my purpose in life; it was my weakness.

During this time of confusion, I met a girl who was two years younger than me. She was from an impoverished area of the country, and she came from a humble family. They lived at the edge of the river where most people who don't have full size houses build a smaller home, just to have a place to sleep. When I took her home to see my mother for the first time, my mom said something to me that I will never forget: "Is that what success looks like to you? That is the reason why you wanted to move out of the house, to be on your own and become independent?" She told me, "I respect your choices, but make sure she does not end up pregnant." That's exactly what happened. She got pregnant and a year later my first child, Manuel Jr, was born. I was still in college, and now I had a family of my own to support at the tender age of 22. I was tasked with making tough decisions in my life. After three and a half years of studying computer programming, I had to admit that I had made the wrong choice. With only one semester left to graduate, I dropped out. In reality, I didn't learn anything about computers. I didn't even like computers.

Dropping out was a relief, I knew I was doing the right thing this time. It's never too late to start again, to live a new story or build a new dream. Will today be the day you start living the life you always dreamed of? Will today be the day you start living your life to the fullest? Will today be the day you finally realize you deserve it? I hope today is the day your life will change. The day you start living the life you had always wished you had the courage to live, once you decided to let go of your fears.

A valuable life lesson I learned was always to follow my dreams. Never allow the influence and opinions of others to distract and delay you from reaching your goals. I was back at square one, under more pressure and worse circumstances, but invariably, life continued. The most successful people are those who accept themselves the way they are; mistakes and all. They don't let mistakes define them. They embrace a new opportunity and future.

Now I had a family to support, so I had to work, to do whatever I had to do to support my them. My mother always told me, "If you are brave enough to have kids, you should be a man enough to support yourself and your family." My mother did just that. She stopped supporting me, so I began working two jobs. I worked in the morning in the governor's office and I worked the overnight shift in a gas station. It was a difficult time for me. I was just 22 with a son and wife to support. I didn't have a clue what I was doing and didn't know how to get my life back on track. There were moments when I was confused, frustrated and had no desire to continue fighting for my dreams. I married the mother of my son and I was determined to make it work. I didn't want my son to go through the same fatherless life I had. I dedicated the next two years to building our marriage and being there for my son Manuel. I was giving him all the love and attention I had not received from my father.

1998

I was 23 years old working at Burger King. The company brought someone in from another country to show us new methods. I was learning a lot - and in just a short period of time, he became my second mentor, and my professional life began to come together for the first time.

Standout from the Crowd

My life had meaning and purpose. After starting as a team member, I decided to build my career in the fast food industry. To do this, I needed to be different; I needed to be unique. I decided to do several things to set myself apart. When everyone else came into work, they came in when they were scheduled, but I would come to work one hour early and leave one hour later. I studied the company manual to become an expert in operations. I spent time with the people that needed me the most instead of running the other way and avoiding them. When my boss thought about completing a task, I had already completed it. If he had to make the schedule, I already had it made, ready for him to verify. If he needed to make the food order, I had already made it for him.

Each day, I dedicated myself to becoming better than I was the day before. In a short period, my success was assured. Every employee in the restaurant was engaged, and I became the manager's right-hand man. Even other employees were happy with my work and had great things to say about me. It made me work harder. And I did, I worked harder and quickly experienced a measure of success as a young adult. Within a few years, I worked my way up in the fast food industry. In a one-year period of time, I went from team member to a successful restaurant general manager. A few months later, I was promoted to a district manager. I oversaw all the restaurants on the northern side of the country. I was doing well in my career and financially. I was making decent money, even more than many doctors in my country.

"There is no growth without change. You've got to let go of some of the old stuff. Often when you're experiencing the most pain, you realize it's coming from trying to control everything or resisting the changes that come with progress. But then you see that light. That beautiful next level and when that is what you have to focus on, incredible things happen."

Decisions Affect Your Destiny

On the other hand, my home life was not so good. My wife and I were different, and we didn't think alike. I had different values, different beliefs than she did. Altogether, my wife and I had been together for over two years. In the beginning, we had an amazing relationship. We had fun, and I learned a lot from her. She was so full of joy and passion, but, to me, it was just fun. I had never thought about getting married. At one point, I took her to spend a week at my mother's house. Even though my father was not in my life, he gave me his last name and made me his son. During that week, my father showed up and he said to me: "Manny, you and her are different, I do not see you marrying a woman like her."

During this time, I had much resentment toward my father and for what he had done. I ended up not taking his advice and we moved in together. When we first moved in together, we were not married, but after my son was born, I realized we would be together forever, so we went ahead and got married. My entire family did not agree with this decision and they were disappointed. At the time, I didn't understand why they were so disappointed. I asked my mother, "Remember that we come from a humble family, why can't I be married to a humble woman?" She never answered my question, but I would soon learn the reason why.

One morning, as I was leaving the house, I kissed my wife and son goodbye. I asked my wife if she wanted to go out to have dinner after work, which was going to be around 9 pm. She agreed. I went off to work in Santiago, about a two-hour drive from home. At the end of the day, I was exhausted from a hard day at work. Before I got home, I had to pass by one of my Burger Kings in my hometown, there is no way around it. I was looking at the drive-thru and the dining room I noticed how full the place was. I looked at my watch, and it was 8:00 pm. I thought, I still have one hour before I need pick my wife up for dinner, so I went inside to help my team. The restaurant was so busy that I lost track of time, and by the time I was able to look at my watch, it was already 10:00 pm. I thought, "oh my God the dinner!" So, I immediately rushed to my apartment, it was only one block away from Burger King.

When I arrived, I opened the door, and my son Manuel Jr. ran to hug me. He yelled "Dad!" Every time I saw my son, I was happy. He was the reflection of me, and, most importantly, I wanted to make sure I was there for him. I tried to be the best father I could be. As I was looking down at him, being careful to make sure he did not fall since he recently had foot surgery and could barely walk. I looked up, and I saw my wife. To my surprise, she stood there with a gun in her hands, pointing it at me. At that moment my entire life flashed before my eyes in a matter of seconds. I didn't know what to do, so I just froze. The time seemed to pass by in slow motion. Then I heard her say "you're going to die today." At that point, I heard the gunshots: one after another. I thought she shot me. Immediately, I let go of my son and rushed to disarm her. I was nervous, and my body was shaking. I really thought it was the last time I'd see my son. Fortunately, I didn't die that night. The two shots had passed my ear, which made my eyes ring for three days. Despite what had happened, she and I tried to work on our marriage. In the end, I realized we were too different, and we were not meant to be together. At that point my son was two years old. We finally decided to separate. We both agreed that I would have custody of our son.

That day I sat down to reflect on my life. At this stage of life, I felt I had committed many mistakes and didn't have much success to show for all my efforts. I recalled all the important events of my life. How I had dropped out of the seminary without taking the vows. Then, how I had dropped out of college without earning a degree. And now, I had a failed marriage. I had nothing to show for all the years of hard work, and now I was a single father with an infant son to support. I began asking myself questions. It seemed evident that I was making the wrong decisions and taking my life in the wrong direction. I had allowed the influence of others to determine the course of my life and my future. Thinking about all of this got me upset. I realized that, "this is my life!" Why am I allowing others to choose my future? That day I decided to take control of my destiny. Moving forward, I would not allow anyone to determine my future. After that day I started a new chapter in my life. My life was great. I was stable, and things were in order to best care for my son.

When You Know, You Know

One afternoon I was sitting at a table inside of one of my restaurants providing some coaching to the restaurant general manager Melissa when a woman opened the door to walk in. She was the most beautiful woman I had ever seen. She was the woman I had always dreamed of, the one I was waiting for my entire life. The moment I saw her I knew she was the woman with whom I wanted to spend the rest of my life. Her name was Fatima. In the next couple weeks, I found out where she worked and sent her flowers every day for three months. She finally agreed to go out with me, and within a few months, we were married. Fatima became my second wife, and within a year, our daughter, Maite, was born. Maite's birth was the culmination of happiness, hope, and joy in our lives. During this time, I felt I had now achieved a certain level of success. I gave myself the opportunity to make it happen again. I believed in me. I didn't allow my past events to determine my life and how I wanted to live. My friends and family were telling me that after my past experiences, I should not trust women, I should not believe in love and I should give up on my dream of having a stable family and being successful at the same time, but I did not listen.

"Each of us must confront our own fears; we must come face to face with them. How we handle our fears will determine where we go with the rest of our lives. We will either experience our life's greatest success and accomplishment or we will be limited by the fear of it."

This time I decided that I was not going to allow anyone to manage my life. I was determined to make my own decisions for the first time. I decided to continue believing in people, in women, in friendships and most importantly believe in myself. It was a key to success. I was 25 years old. I built a beautiful family with Fatima, Manuel Jr, and Maite. Honestly, I was living my dream. I was comfortable with what I had achieved, but in the back of my mind, there was a thorn of doubt. Was I living up to my full potential? I was already thinking, "Is this it?" I was scared about how things were going well for me since I left the seminar up until now.

Give Up to Go Up

Fatima brought so much joy to my life: I enjoyed every second we were together, but at the same time, I was thinking ahead, thinking about what will be within five years. I was wondering what new heights I would reach in the next five years. That answer would come in the form of my first mentor with an urgent message he had for me. Somehow, I feared success. I didn't believe good things can happen to me. After experiencing many setbacks and heartbreaks over time, you can become conditioned to only expect the worst of every situation. Life is full of hills and valleys. What I've learned throughout these years is that every event in your life has a meaning. Embrace every moment as an opportunity to grow. There are no good or bad things in life, only your perspective of them. Once you change the way you look at things your life will change drastically.

2001

One morning in April of 2001, I was working at the restaurant in Burger King in San Francisco. It was a typical day like any other. I was preparing to drive to La Vega, another city on the north side of the country to visit some restaurants but before leaving I was speaking with the manager providing her with instructions. Suddenly, my first mentor, the priest John came to visit me at the restaurant. The visit itself was unusual, but the look on his face was even more troubling. I had never seen him looking so worried. I knew by the look on his face that something is not right. Thoughts were rushing through my mind so fast, that I began to feel nauseated trying to figure out what happened to bring him here. We sat down to talk. He informed me that he had an important message for me. The urgency and the look on his face caused me some concern. I did not know what was going on, but I was sure this was not a routine visit. As we were sitting down in the dining room to talk, he immediately said: "Manny, it is time for you to leave the country."
I am not sure if I heard right! I asked, "Why do I need to leave?"
I mean..., I had a great job, a beautiful family, and my mother close by. I've finally reached a level of success. Why should I give all of this up? I asked him, "Why?" He said, "I do not know the answer. The only thing I know is that this morning I was praying, and God told me to tell you that it is time for you to leave the country. We have to get you ready Manny," he said. I was so scared and confused. Here was my mentor, my father figure telling me to give

up all the success that I had achieved, to leave behind everything and everyone including my wife, kids, and mother. I said, "You are the person that always pushed me never to give up; to continue trying until I achieve my goals. I haven't reached my goal here." At that moment I thought he doesn't want me to be good. He knows about all the challenges I have faced and now for the first time in my life I was feeling good about myself and the job I was doing. Now more than ever, my life has meaning. How could he suggest such a thing?

"You taught me to follow my dreams and not to allow anyone to take that from me." I said. Immediately he replied, "Manny it is time for you to move."

We went back and forth for some time. I came up with every argument I could think of. I've never been there! I could not even speak English! I did not have enough money saved to take care of my family and move to another country! No matter the excuse, he was firm on the fact that I had to leave. Before he left, he said, "Manny, you do not have much time. Make sure you make the decision soon." Honestly, I was terrified, scared, I did not know what to think or what to do. I could not sleep that night thinking about the urgent message he delivered. I had major doubts to make another huge mistake. In my short life I had already made so many wrong decisions; I did not want to make another. I was being asked to make a significant decision that didn't seem to make any sense! I did not know if leaving my wife, the love of my life, and my two young children was the right thing to do.

The next morning, I woke up and I sat with my wife prepared to tell her what the priest John told me. She noticed I did not sleep the night before and that I was preoccupied and worried. She knew something was not right, and there was a lot on my mind. At first, she thought that something was happening at work because usually I took the problems at work to my house. With some hesitation in my voice, I told her what John said, and immediately she said: "He is crazy!" Honestly, I did not expect her response to be any different. I needed more answers. Not only for me but also for my wife and my family, so I went to the priests' house that morning seeking more details. However, he had nothing more to tell me. Only the insistence that I had to leave the country as soon as possible. He said, "We need to start getting you prepared with a visa because you have to leave the country as soon as possible." At this point I knew he was serious about it. I also thought maybe someone was trying to kill me! My life was in danger! My family was in danger! There was a lot of different hypotheses that was coming to my mind, but I had to trust him. It was a tough decision to make. I thought it over for couple weeks and eventually decided to start the process to move out of the country. With her heart broken, my wife supported my decision to leave the country. I want to give my mentor the opportunity and follow his directions. I have followed his directions since I was 15 years old and he has demonstrated to me he wants the best for me. Why would this time will be different?

As the time passed and I was getting close to the date of leaving my life behind. I thought about my life and the doubts arrived with a ton of questions that I did not have answers to. What about if I leave everything behind and I am not making the right decision? What about if I stayed and I made the wrong decision? I was confused. I spent many days and nights thinking about the pros and cons, trying to find one excuse not to leave my country and my family behind. It was one of the most difficult decisions that I've had to make in my life at this point, because now it is not only me. I have two children and my wife. On the other hand, I know if I leave the country, I would be fulfilling one of my dreams of going to another country to learn, grow and become a millionaire.

Throughout this process, I saw my reluctance that stemmed from the comfort that I was feeling. I was "playing it safe." I realized that life is a gamble. For me to live to my full potential, I had to take the chance. So, I got a visa. I was ready to leave everything behind; my wife, children, mother, job, home, and start all over again. I did not know how to do it, but I had the gut feeling that I was doing the right thing. I was ready to get out of my comfort zone and face my fears and become successful. This would provide the best life for my family. Who is not willing to do anything possible for their children, to provide a better education, to raise your children in a different environment that you were raised?

His urging message changed the course of my life. Sometimes for your life to change drastically you just need the right person of influence to help push you where you need to go. For me, it was the priest who came to change my life around. Some people have to leave everything behind because their lives are in danger, others for economic reasons and for decisions that have been made for them. In my case, it was a gut feeling from the priest John. I was not sure where I would go. I had some family in Spain from my mother's side and a few friends in the United States. At this point, I knew that I had to go, but I had no idea where? That was the question I needed to answer.

It was September 11, 2001. The terrorist attacks on the World Trade Center in New York City had just taken place. This added another layer of fear and uncertainty, causing me to wonder if I was making the right decision in moving to the United States or Spain. But God had plans for me. I continued with my preparations to leave the country. During this time, I received a visit from my mentor John's brother. He was visiting from the United States. He had been living there for the past ten years where he was a chef at a prestigious restaurant in New Jersey. He had a proposition for me. He wanted to start a business, buying and running a supermarket in New York City. He was looking for someone to manage the supermarket for him. As he was telling his brother about his plans, his brother told him of my upcoming move outside of the Dominican Republic, and that I would be the perfect person for the job. With that in mind, he came to my office to offer me a 50/50 partnership in his new business venture. It sounded amazing! He said that I would be making around five thousand dollars each month, back then this was a lot of money. His proposition was the sign I needed to decide on where to move. I went home and discussed it with my wife, and the arrangement sounded like a perfect solution for me. It was very hard for Fatima. She cried a lot that night and almost every day, realizing that we would be separated for some time while I would be in another country securing our future. However, the decision had been made, and this seemed like an answer to our prayers. With this offer, I was sure that I had made the right decision and I would be secure when I moved to the U.S. I went out the next morning and purchased my airline ticket. I would be leaving on October 21, 2001.

That morning finally came, and it was difficult to leave my family. My wife was crying, and my children were clinging to me, but I had to make the sacrifice to provide a better future for us. As a child, I saw people that went to the United States and returned home within a year, successful and RICH! I thought to myself, "Why should I be any different?" That morning, the priest John came to take me to the airport. I cried the entire way holding on to my wife's hand. Even though I kept asking myself, "Why am I doing this? Because the priest had a dream? What if I'm making a huge mistake?" However, the arrangements were already made, and with a heavy heart, I left behind everything I knew and loved.

Our life is the subtotal of decisions we make or failed to make. We need to be willing to take the chance, to take the risk and to make the necessary sacrifices. People are not willing to give up their comfort and replace it with uncomfortable moments to create outstanding lives. I made wrong decisions that took me through painful experiences in my life, but I understand we all have a birth and expiration date attached to our lives. The only thing that matters is the journey in between. The journey represents what impact you make while you are here.

Will others say you lived or just existed? I recently watched one of Pixar's latest movies "Coco" with my family. I mean we watched it over and over and over for a whole week. Each time I was able to pick up on some very cool and deep concepts that made me think about my life. One being the "Final Death." That concept originates from traditional Mexican ideology of "three deaths." The three deaths include:

- Physical – Death of the body
- Natural - Returned to nature's cycle
- Final Death – You disappear into thin air after no one remembers you

The "final death" really hit home for me. I immediately started thinking about how I wanted to be remembered. Thus far in my life, I had allowed others to make decisions for me. How many of you have done the same thing? Think about it… Whenever you do not decide you hand over the power of your life to someone else. I call it "living by default." To be successful, you must live life by design. This means to take control of your life by having enough guts to decide the direction you want it to go. History remembers the risk takers. Will you stop playing it safe for a chance to live forever in the hearts and minds of those who's path you have crossed? You matter, your legacy matters, just decide and separate yourself from the outcome.

According to some recent research, the average adult makes about 35,000 remotely conscious decisions every day. Each person is different depending on the level of responsibility they hold. Sounds crazy right? We make 226 decisions each day on just food alone according to researchers at Cornell University. You see, there are too many decisions in a day to leave it up to chance. There are also too many variables that affect your decisions. One of them being your environment or upbringing. You learned earlier about my background, now I will be showing you how I transitioned to a better life. It doesn't matter where you came from, or how-to severe childhood has been. It doesn't even matter how late you start in life. What does matter is, how bad you want it. Let me ask you; How much you are willing to sacrifice to achieve your goals?

There comes a time in life where a choice must be made that will determine your future. Success always moves forward. You're either growing or dying. Before you move to the other side to your greatness, a transition must take place. That transition for me was painful. I had to go against everything and almost everyone I knew to break away from a way of thinking that stunted my growth. Let me tell you. It is a process, and you must be extraordinarily patient and mentally tough to withstand the resistance to change. This transition has three phases for me:

Overcome your fear of failure – The battle begins and ends in the mind, so the first thing you must do is detach yourself from any limiting people or beliefs from your past. Surround yourself with positive people that inspire and challenge norms that you are accustomed to. You must forgive yourself; you need to understand that you can make mistakes, that you can fail many times, that you do not have to be perfect to be good, that you do not need to know everything.

Visualize the life you want - If you can imagine it in your head, you can have it in your life. Whatever you do, don't ever stop dreaming. Set goals, make plans and take massive action. If you do not see it in your mind, you will not see it in real life. You must close your eyes and see yourself having this dream, touch it, feel it.

Fully commit yourself - Once you decide to move forward, make sure to burn the bridge down that you just crossed so going back won't be an option. To make your commitment stick, you must have a strong "Why" that will continuously fuel you on your journey. I believe a commitment to ourselves is the most critical part of the process. Most of the time, we are not committed to our desires. Have you decided you are going to lose weight and you start changing your habits the first week, and things are going well, but the following week you dropped. Sometimes we decide to read a book for 30 minutes every day: We get excited to go to the library purchase a few books, within couple days you find yourself giving excuses not to read the book.

Everyone will have a unique experience and journey. One thing for sure is there will be obstacles along the journey that will take you far out of your comfort zone. And you will not recognize yourself at times. Your brain will go into shock because it is designed to keep you comfortable and calm. You will encounter pain you've never felt before. Your lows will be very low, pushing you to the brink, but you will persevere because you have to. Just like I had to. Did you forget that you burned the bridge to go back home? The only option now is to give up or rise to another level.

My journey began with the end in mind. I could smell the land of the free and taste the opportunities waiting for me in America almost seventeen years ago. I don't know how, but I know my life was not going to be the same after I moved to the United States.

Every decision counts. Will you always make the right decision? Of course not. No one is perfect, but each time that you step outside your comfort zone and make the tough calls, you grow stronger and wiser. That experience gives you a competitive advantage personally and professionally. Think about it: You will not find someone that has achieved success sitting, waiting for things to happen. They constantly move out of their comfort zone. They constantly challenge themselves to be better than the day before. They're willing to sacrifice and not allow anyone's opinion to destroy their dream.

There are only two people in this world. Those who call the shots and those who take orders. And that truth has been made clear in every phrase possible: "Those who talk and those who walk, those who want to be and those who be." It's a simple lesson. Make decisions or take orders. Either way, you win because you took the initiative to choose your destiny.

Moving to the United States was not an easy decision to make. I had it all planned, and it wasn't supposed to be difficult. But just because we plan it, doesn't mean it always works out that way. What I'm about to share with you in the next few chapters are the most uncomfortable moments of my life. How I went from being homeless to a successful businessman? I was lucky I found someone who taught me the secret of success. These are the methods I learned in my first ten years in the United States, and I am excited to share with you.

Never Give Up on Your Dreams

2001

Just Do It Anyway

October 21, 2001: The day had finally come. My bags were packed and loaded into the trunk of the car ready to take me to the airport away from everything I knew and loved. I was on the way to the airport with my wife and children to see me off. I had mixed feelings. There was still doubt and fear to overcome, and deep sadness in leaving my family. I was still questioning my decision, and the mixed emotions made me feel very vulnerable. It was a strange feeling; I was not sure if I was doing the right thing or not, I knew I would be missing my wife and kids, my family, friends, even the people that I worked with. During this moment, so many things came to my mind. I was so confused, I was sad, and I was not feeling good about the decision that I had made, but I still chose to move forward. I knew it would be difficult to be in a country not knowing anyone and not speaking their language but even with that I took the risk.

I will never forget how far I have come. All the obstacles, sadness and setbacks; all the times that I kept pushing on even when I felt I could not do it. All the moments when things did not happen the way I planned, and I still tried until it was completed. All the mornings that I did not want to wake up to go to work and I still did. All the times that I just wanted to give up my dreams, but I went through another day and all rejections when people did not believe in me, and I still did it. The most important of all were the strengths I obtained in the process from my failures.

Dreams can become a reality only if you are willing to move out of your comfort zone. I kept repeating this over and over because I knew there was no other way to be happy and achieve success in life.

During the morning drive to the airport, I became hyper-sensitive of everything I passed on the roads. I looked at my surroundings and thought, would I ever see my country again? I was holding my son and baby daughter and wondering when I would see them again. I looked at my wife and thought of all the beautiful moments we shared together. I remembered every event that happened in our lives: the moment I first met her and just knew she was the woman I wanted as my wife for the rest of my life. I was so determined to win her heart. How magical our relationship was, and how complete we felt when our daughter Maite was born. I thought about the trips we sometimes took to the beach we had such fun times together. How could I leave that all behind? I looked at the palm trees, the beautiful green mountains, and felt the hot tropical sun kiss my skin. I saw the people on the streets and fell in love for my culture and country for the first time. Honestly, all the things I hated in the past I started paying attention to and they were suddenly beautiful to me at this moment. I noticed that sometimes we don't value things until they are in jeopardy. It was so painful leaving, but I had made up my mind to leave and work at building an even better life for myself and my family. I knew if I stayed in my country, I would not be able to achieve much success. Soon I will be one more, part of the 95 percent of the people that are just living paycheck to paycheck. I was motivated by the desire to learn from others that already achieved what I want to achieve. I was open to learning anything and everything - and I looked forward to it. Life goes on whether you choose to move on and take a chance in the unknown or stay behind, looking in your past, thinking about of what could've been.

When I was to board the airplane, I said my goodbyes and knew I could not turn around to look at them. If I did, I would not be able to leave my country. My wife Fatima and I were crying, and my kids were looking on, anxious and confused. I kissed them goodbye, hugged my wife and embraced the priest, John, one last time before I departed. While I was saying my goodbyes, I kept thinking to myself, "I will be back in a year rich and successful." That thought helped me to be strong. So, as I started to walk to the gate, I did not look back. All I heard was crying from my wife and children echoing in my ears. I was sad and scared during that three-hour flight to New

York. I cried the entire time. I was barely out of the country, and I missed them. I had to succeed for them. While I was looking at the sky 36,000-feet above the ground I started thinking about all things that I needed to accomplish, and I began to feel some excitement. I thought back to my childhood impressions of comfortable living and wealth to be found in the United States. There was no doubt in my mind that I would make it. I thought, at this stage of my life I have learned so much from my failures, if others got rich in one year, I could do it in six months. I had it all planned in my mind. I thought it would be so easy to become rich in the United States. I was not worried about learning English or having a superior education. Everyone knows America is the land of opportunity, but what I did not know back then was that the real America was a bit different than advertised. The priest John had arranged me to stay with an old friend and his wife until the supermarket was purchased and I could start working in my new adventure. When we spoke a few weeks before, he was very kind and told me that I could stay with them as long as I needed. I was so happy that he was able to open his house for me and was allowing me to stay with his family. I cannot believe that everything was lining up for me. First, the priest's brother and now my friend would allow me to stay at his house. What can go wrong, I thought.

Turn Setbacks into Stepping Stones

Going through immigration at the airport, the official asked me a few questions and my only responses were yes or no. At the time, I didn't know any English: just two words "yes" and "no." He was frustrated to the point that he told me to go. He even had to make gestures for me to understand I was clear to go. I was a little bit ashamed that someone wanted to speak with me and I was not able to communicate. That was the first time I experienced that feeling. It was horrible knowing that I didn't have control over my life.

On October 21, 2001 my friend came that night to pick me up from Kennedy International Airport in New York City. I walked out of the terminal to meet him, and we laughed and exchanged hugs. It was comforting to see a familiar face from home. Getting into the car I looked down at the pavement, and to my surprise there was a $20 bill. I thought to myself, "Oh my God, it is true! There is money laying in the streets here in America." In my ignorance, I did not pick up the money. I thought, "I will start picking up money tomorrow." Little did I know the hardships that awaited. Feeling some of my doubts and fears recede, I happily took in the sights of the city. I was amazed and impressed by the buildings, lights, cars, and cold weather. These attractions were all new experiences for me. I had never seen anything like this before, and the excitement of New York City helped me to forget more of my fears and misgivings for a little bit. During this tour of Manhattan, I was fascinated with the entire city. I was almost overwhelmed with the massive skyscrapers, yellow taxicabs, and so many people in winter jackets rushing around. We stopped for a few minutes to see another old friend. He had a portable stand selling coffee in the street. I thought to myself, "How could he be so stupid to be selling coffee when there are so many better opportunities to make money here in the land of the opportunity?"

During the tour, he was giving me advice on the "dos" and "don't" about the city, the people, the laws, the police, and more. He also was telling me what happened with a few of our mutual friends that were in jail for doing illegal activities. In this moment while he was telling me about why my friends went to jail, I realized to become rich would not be so easy because I was not willing to sell drugs or do any illegal activity to put myself and others at risk. He also showed me how Manhattan is divided into three sides: downtown is where the rich people live, uptown is where the poor people live, and midtown is where the middle-class people live. I was impressed, in my country everyone lived together you can have some areas better than others, but the division was not that noticeable. Finally, he said, "Let's go home to have something to eat. My wife is making dinner for us. I said, "I am hungry, I have not eaten anything all day plus I want to call back home and share with my wife how beautiful is New York City and how my friends are taking care of me. As we arrived at his apartment the dinner was ready and waiting for us. I met his wife and she was very nice but not as friendly as I expected. I did not think much about it, and we sat down and ate dinner and drank a few beers. We were catching up on all our life experiences. After we finished eating, he invited me up to the roof to see the view of the city. I went happily, feeling comfortable and reliving memories of our time together back home. I was at ease and enjoying myself. We were up there for about an hour, and he seemed to get more uncomfortable as time went on. I wondered what the problem was when he turned to me and delivered some unexpected news. He said, "Manny, I am sorry that I have to tell you this, but I spoke with my wife earlier, and she says that you cannot stay here with us. She does not know you, and she does not feel comfortable with a strange man in the house. You have to find another place to stay. I hope you understand; I have my hands tied."

I was shocked. Couldn't he have told me this before I came? Now it's almost 11 p.m., where should I go? Whom should I call? I can understand his wife's feeling, but had I known, I could have made other arrangements. However, I had no choice but to leave his house. Feeling surprised and a little disgruntled, I told him, "Okay, I will stay tonight, and in the morning, I will find someplace to go". He said, "You can stay, but not inside the apartment. You can stay downstairs in a little room by the dumpster area. I can give you a pillow and a blanket, so you will not be too cold." I could not believe what I was hearing. My first night in this new country, the beginning of the rest of my life, the land of the opportunity and I had to sleep on the ground by a dumpster? I thought it was a joke, but as he led me downstairs, I realized it was all too real.

That night while I was laying on the cold hard floor, I couldn't believe this was happening. I had my head in my hands, sitting in a small storage room with the discarded pieces of other people's lives. I was surrounded by old pictures, dusty equipment, and broken furniture and couple mice around me. I struggled with my feelings trying not to feel as discarded as the old items around me. During this night I hardly slept. I started thinking about what just happened. I was trying to process what was going on with people in this country. I don't think I would do the same to anyone if I was in my country. All my doubts and fears came crashing down. All I could think was that I'd made the biggest mistake of my life! I thought, "God, why is this happening to me?" I considered going back home: My first night in the United of States and I already failed. I thought if this is my first night, how are the rest going to play out. The only problem was I had already quit my job. I really did not want to go back home to hear everyone say, "I told you so." I didn't want them to see me as a failure, or a loser. I had not even called my wife; I didn't want to listen to her say "I told you so." So, that night I told myself I could figure something out until the business partnership in the supermarket got started.

Through hours of thinking, I decided not to complain. I would take the necessary steps to make my dreams a reality. I stopped making excuses and began thinking about possible solutions to my problems. I had already overcome many obstacles in my life. At the time, I thought those situations were insurmountable. However, looking back I realized I was being prepared for the rest of my life. It was the best thing that could have happened to me. I said to myself, "In a year, this will all be over, and I will look back and realize how easy everything was." I just needed to find a solution to my problems. Once I figured out how to overcome this obstacle, it will become possible and real.

During tough moments we need to be strong, happy, thankful, and appreciative of what we have. We must realize this moment will pass, the morning will come, and we will live another day. The morning will bring a new opportunity to fight for what we want to accomplish. It's easy to show happiness, to feel good, to be strong and have faith when things are going great, and everything is going your way. The real test is to be steadfast during the hard times. This is the time when you need to show how bad you want to achieve your goals. Be happy and understand everything happens to you is for a reason.

At that moment I learned things don't always happen the way we plan and how we expect them to. I realized things happen how they need to happen. It is a necessary lesson to develop you into the person you need to become. Challenging times help you identify and understand   your strengths and weakness. So, that night I decided to take this event as a positive and understand that everything has a purpose. I may not be able to see the reason right now, but I know I will be able to see it later. I also learned when we have difficult times in life is when we have to stay positive and show that you can be happy and grateful. With this clarity, I finally fell asleep. The next morning, I woke up with more energy, convinced I would change my life around by any means necessary to create a better future. I knew what I wanted, and when I wanted it. I did not care if I had to work 20 hours a day, sleep in the park, under a bridge, or eat from a trash can. No matter what, I would accomplish my dreams.

I called the priest's brother, my new business partner. I explained what just happened and I asked for advice. He listened to it all and then told me to catch a bus to his home in Bricktown, New Jersey. Imagine, I did not speak any English and being from the tropics, I didn't even have a winter coat It was late October in New York City, and I had to venture out on my own. I made my way to the Port Authority Bus Terminal on 42 street in New York with all my belongings. As I entered, I realized it was huge and completely overwhelming I wondered how I would find the right bus. I was very intimidated, but I didn't have a choice. I entered what appeared to be a maze. Flashing signs everywhere, a voice over the speaker I could not understand and hundreds of people running in every direction. I wondered why everyone was in such a hurry. As I was looking around, I saw a young man cleaning the floors. He looked Hispanic, so I approached him and asked for help. He was very kind. He even helped me to buy my ticket and showed me where to go to find the right bus. Feeling relieved, I started the ride to Bricktown, but realized I didn't know where to get off. Luckily, the man next to me was getting off at the same stop, so I followed him. Gratefully, I was able to find my contact waiting for me.

I was intending on salvaging my pride and securing my future. I was ready to start our partnership, but he was still working out the details of the purchase. He lived in a charming, upper-class neighborhood - and I lived in his basement for a couple of weeks, doing odd jobs around his house while he worked on closing the deal for the supermarket. I asked him for details and a timeframe to start our working partnership. I wanted to put the bad start behind me and get on the road to becoming successful. He had been a little distant in his attitude, and I was anxious to start working. After about two weeks, I sat down with him and asked what was happening. "I have already been here in America for a few weeks, and I still haven't worked. I need to send money home to my family, and I do not feel comfortable living on your charity." He looked me straight in the eye and asked me to go outside for a walk with him. Once he said that to me, I felt there was something wrong. It reminded of my experience with my other friend in New York. I could feel the same bubbling. It was a gut-wrenching sensation. As we were walking, he explained to me how deals were made in the USA. He told me he made an offer on the supermarket. I didn't understand anything, but I was happy he made an offer. This meant things were coming along, I thought. In my country, if you have the money, you purchased the property. As we were walking, he delivered the heartbreaking news that created another massive setback in my life. He said, "The deal fell through. I could not buy the business, so there is no supermarket for you to run. Someone won the bid on the property." He also told me that I needed to move to another area that I could afford and find a job to support myself.

In less than four weeks I experienced two huge setback in my life. I was feeling devastated and felt like crying my heart out. What do you do when nothing is going as planned and you're hit with setback after setback? After a couple of minutes digesting the bad news and looking for a way to get myself back on track, I asked him if he could get me a job in the restaurant where he worked., I knew he was the main chef, so he'd be able to hire his team. He told me, "No, they are not hiring at this time." He also said, "I think you should get your stuff and go. I know a place that is renting a room. I am sure in Lakewood you will find a job. There are many immigrants in that town."

As we drove to my new home, the houses and neighborhoods were getting worse and worse. I had not seen a neighborhood like that before. I didn't think there were such places in America. I thought everyone had money and lived in beautiful homes and drove expensive cars. How could anyone be unfortunate in the land of opportunity? In my ignorance, I thought if there was money for immigrants to become productive and successful, how could any American be poor? At that moment I had not realized how difficult it was to become successful in America. The houses were old and rundown. There was garbage in the yards and on the streets. The roads were full of potholes, and there were people of all colors roaming the streets. I could tell some were homeless, drunk, or high on something. We ended up in Lakewood, New Jersey. He finally stopped at a house and told me to wait in the car. I was scared as people looked at me while I waited. As others were looking at me, I was looking at him, approaching the house. A woman opened the door, and they spoke for a few minutes. I realized he already had planned everything. He came back to the car and told me it was all arranged. I would be renting a room here for $125 per month, and I needed to pay the landlady the first month right now. At this point, I had only $300 to my name. I had no choice. I paid for the room and went inside to see my new home. To say that I was shocked would be an understatement. It was not a room I had just rented. It was a walk-in closet. It had no furniture, not even a bed. All I had was the clothes on my back. As I toured the house, she explained to me that there was no heat or air conditioning. The carpet was old, dirty and had a strange smell. She showed me the bathroom I had to share with people I didn't know. While we walked through the entire house, I thought it was strange when I noticed there were beds throughout every room in the house, even the garage, except for my room. At the time, I did not know what it meant. It was not long before I found out.

I went into my closet and while I was sitting on the floor with my hands on my head thinking about what had just happened. Just a month ago, I was with my family in my apartment, with a great job in an environment I loved. Now I'm in a strange country surrounded by people I had never seen in my life. If you can think about an uncomfortable situation, this has been the most uncomfortable situation in my entire life. I felt miserable, defeated, insecure and lost. At that point, I did not know what to do. I did not have a job and was almost out of money. I had two children and wife who were waiting for me to send money. I sat down for hours crying saying horrible things about myself. How stupid I was, in that moment I realized all my friends and my family were right, I am stupid.

Trust but Verify

In my first couple of months in America, I learned that I needed to trust others, but I also needed to verify for myself first. I still believe in people. I think that in order for us to achieve any level of success in life we must work together with others. There are individuals who are going to help you succeed in your journey. We must trust ourselves and others. I stood in my new home and took a hard look at my situation. This was just another new challenge in my life, and I had to stay positive and motivate myself. I was not willing to give up. I would do whatever it took to rise out of this situation. I remember my mother always used to say, *"In every bad situation, something good comes out of it."* At that point, I was waiting for anything good to come out of this situation. I still had a family back home to support. I didn't have the luxury of giving up. As evening fell, I began hearing more and more voices in the house. Many more than the Mexican family that rented me the closet. I went into the kitchen and was amazed at the sight that greeted me. Seventeen people were in there, some were sitting on the table, others were standing having dinner. At first, I thought she sold food as a side hustle, but a few minutes later I realized they had rented living space to all these people. That is why there were beds everywhere. I was now living with 17 people I did not know. I didn't know where they came from or even if they were decent people. We were all living together in a cold house because the heat did not work.

So, here I was, an illegal immigrant, with no job. I did not speak the language, had very little money, and on top of all that, lived in and overcrowded house. Could things get any worse? I tried very hard not to sink into despair. With so little money left, there were days that I was eating out of the trash until I found a job. As time passed, and since I was a stranger in this country, these people became my new friends. They were all I really had. They were nice and hardworking, but they had no ambition or desire to achieve anything in life. They drank every day, used drugs and what made matters worse, they came with little to no education. It was a very dysfunctional environment to be in.

At this moment, I did not have anyone to rely on, anyone whom I could count on. I had no one to call, or any family to talk to. I was completely lost. I did not know where to start, what to do, and how to do it. I was here living with 17 people but at the same time alone. I was from a different race. We all spoke the same language, but I was from the Caribbean and they were from Mexico and South

America. I knew that I needed to do something, so I started talking to all of them. I was trying to understand what they do, but most importantly I was trying to get a job. I found out they worked in a variety of jobs: landscaping, construction, factories, and housekeeping. I was amazed of how content they were to make just enough money to pay the bills and have enough left over to buy alcohol. Most of them woke up early every morning to wait in the streets until someone picked them up for day labor. As I was asking everyone for help to get a job in the same place they were working, I received "no" for an answer from everyone. At that moment, I asked myself "what is wrong with everyone here?" Nobody is willing to help you, everyone only thought about themselves. For years I complained about the people in my country because some people were selfish but once I experienced this, I thought we were not that bad after all. You cannot imagine how uncomfortable I felt. I could not believe what I had done to my life and my future. If I'm completely honest with you, once I was in that house, I lost all hope for my dreams. I cried almost every day. I did not want to call my wife to tell her about the big mistake I had made. I had failed in so many ways in life. I could not call my ex-boss to tell him I screwed up and I wanted my job back. I knew at this point things were not going to work the way I planned. I was scared. I didn't know what to do and what to expect any more in life. What else can go wrong? This had been my life. My father rejected me, I dropped out of seminary, I dropped out of college, and I failed in my first marriage, almost losing my life in the process. Now, when I thought I saw a light at the end of the tunnel, I ended up in an uncomfortable situation, in a stranger country, with people who had no ambition, no education, in the middle of drugs and alcohol and most important I left my kids and the love of my life behind Fatima.

Throughout the process, I felt the priest set me up for failure. He had come to this country before, so he knew how things were here. He said our mutual friends would help me in New York, but I did not receive any assistance. I felt alone and abandoned by everyone. Everything I was banking on fell through the cracks and left me on my own in a distant land. I was not sure if the priest John wanted to give a life lesson or wanted me dead. I began to blame everyone else for my failures. I thought I was doing what everyone normally did, but, the only person who was hurt was me. Eventually I was able to shake it off, reflect and recharge. It took time, but it came around.

The next day, I woke up committed to becoming successful. I was trying to be positive, to have hope. I was not willing to give up after coming across a few obstacles. It was difficult to be positive, but I did not have any other choice. I went for a walk down the street and looked at people waiting on the corner. There were about 20 other Hispanic immigrants. As I was walking, I saw a car stop and pick up one of the guys. I approached one of the men I had recognized from home, and I asked: "What are you doing here?" He told me he was a "*Jornalero*," and I replied, "What is a *Jornalero* mean?". He then said its when people like me who do not have a job and are an illegal in this country, we stop here every morning waiting for people to stop by and pick us up when they need any help in cleaning their houses, maintenance, and more. We do everything and anything. He also said, the beauty of this job is we work when we want, we do not have a boss, and we do not pay taxes. Wow. I thought. I did not leave everything behind to work to pay the bills. I want something more significant for me. As I saw an opportunity for me to make some money. I was clear this would be only temporary. I did not want to be one of them for the rest of my life. I did not want to fall in the same tramp. As we continued with the conversation, I asked him another question. How do you get paid? He said, "We get paid cash, and we agree before we leave here but sometimes, we do the job and end up not getting paid a dime for the labor. It is a risk we take, but we do not have any other way to make money.

I was cold because I did not have a jackct to wcar, but I staycd there. It was going to be my new life. Every time a car stopped all the guys ran after the car to be the person who was picked. It was depressing observing how you get picked and how you beg for someone to pick you. After the day was over, I couldn't feel my hands. They were frozen from the cold weather. I went back home. I knew I had to be a jornalero if I wanted to survive in this country. I needed to make some money and here was an opportunity for me to make some money. As the days passed, I had only one meal a day. I wanted to save money. I remember going to a Chinese restaurant every day to order chicken wings and pork rice. That was my diet for months. The employees knew me within a week and knew exactly what I was ordering. Every morning I woke up early to stop in the streets waiting for someone to pick me up like everyone else. We were fighting to get into the car every time someone stopped. I still didn't have a jacket to wear in the cold winter of New Jersey and that circumstances made it more uncomfortable. There were times I spent the entire day there, and no one picked me. It was depressing. Also, the people I was living with did not help at all; they only were working to pay their bills and have money for beer and drugs. They did not have dreams like me. As the time was passed, I started looking for different type of job. I did not want to depend on what the day would bring me. I had a family back in the Dominican Republic and they were expecting me to support them. In the meanwhile, I was lying to my wife. I was telling her that things were great for me. I was getting my feet on the ground and soon I would be sending money. I think she knew things were not good for me, as much as I tried to hide it from her. She could feel it in my tone of my voice.

There were also many times that I had to go to the Church to get free clothes and food because I could not get steady work. I became a refugee, one of the poorest people in society. It was so painful - an incredible challenge for me, wearing dirty clothes, walking in the cold weather in New Jersey for miles. However, I still had dreams. I knew that one day, I would be able to succeed.

Over the next few months, I tried to stay positive, but my "American Dream" had turned into a nightmare. I went out and got two jobs, working in fast-food restaurants, starting at the very bottom because I could not speak English. I tried to stay motivated, knowing I was willing to work hard for a better future. Reality hit me, and I started to realize I would not find success and be able to return home to my family in a year as I had promised. To become successful and wealthy would take much longer than one year. I was not willing to go back without achieving what I had promised. I was not prepared to live without my wife for that long, so I would have to ask her to come to America. Every day, on my way to work I would see nice cars driving by, families with their children, parents taking their kids to school and always I thought about my family, knowing that one day they would be here with me. I promised myself one day, I would drive an expensive car like theirs. I would have a beautiful house and take my kids to the park to play. One day finally my wife will be here with me, next to me.

How could I ask my wife Fatima to leave our daughter with her family, so she could be here with me? I didn't want to bring my children here to live in my current situation, so they would have to stay on the island with our family. I didn't even have a decent job so that I could afford to move to an apartment. It was a difficult decision for her to make. We had many conversations before she made her decision to move here with me. Once she arrived in the states, I was so happy, finally one good thing happened to me. I remember her face when she got into the house for the first time, she looked in my face and asked, "This is why you left everything behind?" Honestly, I was devastated. By now, I was used to the life having been there for three months already. She was scared and confused. Her heart was divided in two. On one side, she was happy to be with me, but at the same time she was missing our kids and her family. She experienced the same feeling as me, she was disappointed in me.

I remember at the end of the year I found a job at Burger King. I had to wake up every morning at 4am, walk for about three miles to catch the bus to be at work at 5am. One morning there was a snowstorm, the temperature was well below freezing. I still did not own a winter jacket, so I had to walk three miles in a snowstorm to catch the bus. Hesitating to walk in the snow with the lower temperature. I thought about asking Robert, one of the guys that lived with me in the house, to take me to the bus stop. He had a car and every day he passed me on his way to going to work. So I did exactly that. "Hey Robert, can you please drop me off at the bus station on your way home? I do not have a jacket and its really cold." He replied, "I am sorry but today I will be taking a different route." So, at once I started walking to the bus stop and within a few minutes I started feeling the cold weather. My hands and fingers began to freeze. I did not feel my ears and I couldn't breathe. As I was walking in the snow, I touched my nose as it was numb and the top layer of my skin peeled off. I started thinking about Fatima who was asleep in the house. I thought about my children Manuel Jr. and Maite. I needed to find the energy, the motivation to get to the bus station. As I was getting close, shivering and in agony, I looked at the road, there was one car that was approaching me. I noticed it was Robert who just keep riding by. Luckily, my entire body was so frozen, I could not process how wrong he did me. A couple years later I gave Robert a life lesson that I am sure he would never forget. He came to me one day to help him get a job. I knew that I was his last hope, but despite of how he behaved towards me, I helped him out. I treated him like I wanted to be treated.

Over time, I worked a variety of different jobs, trying to earn enough money to fulfill my dream of becoming successful. Before I knew it, five years had passed. Five years of struggling at low paying jobs and living at the bottom end of society. I was working so hard, but I was not making any progress. I became numb to my dreams and ambitions. I became comfortable. I was another member of the working-class poor… just another face in the crowd. I worked in different factories, Burger King, McDonalds, cleaning carpet, construction, etc. I wasn't getting anywhere in life. This was not what I had left my country for. I lost hope; I was scared for myself, I did not know how to do it. I was afraid to lose the little bit I had conquered. We are only afraid to lose something that we own, but this fear disappears when we understand we born with a purpose and it is our responsibility to find it.

I remember working in landscaping and going to a fast food restaurant for lunch with all my pears. As I was seating in a table there was a family seating eating their burger, once they saw me with my tray going to the table next to them, they stood up and moved to another table, they looked at us with scorn. I knew we were dirty and smelled bad. They looked at me like was a criminal and a lowlife. Nobody was willing to sit near us. I felt so depressed to see how people rejected us. I finally woke up on that day and had enough. I started thinking here I was, living in a house with 17 other people with no ambition. I knew I was better than this and I had to make a change to get back on track. I thought back to my mentor and remembered something he told me years before. He said, "Manny, be careful of the people you hang around and spend time with because you will become just like them without realizing it." He was right. I started to have no ambition just like all the other people that lived in that house. On that day, something was different, I knew something had to change, I realized I had to stop living this way. I did not know how I was going to do it, but I was going to make a change in my life. That day one of the coworkers, Andres, told me It was a wakeup call for me. I had been in America for five years working all types of job trying to succeed but I only received rejections. At the end of the day it had been my fault, I never took any actions, I never found another way to succeed. I stayed with the same methods I learned when I moved to the house.

I realized that if I wanted to change my life, I had to change every aspect: I had to change where I lived; change the people I surrounded myself with; I need to find successful people that have achieved what I wanted to accomplish in life. I was feeling miserable because I had surrounded myself with people who lived miserable lives. I had to accept that I was not perfect and forgive myself for the mistakes that I had made. Once I forgave myself, it gave me the ability to move forward. It is easy to say than do, I did not know anyone that could help me, I did not have enough money to move, and I was not ready to hang out with others with different education than me.

What should I do? I asked myself this question - over and over again. So, I thought I had to make a plan to expose myself to the kind of people that were successful so that I could learn to be like them. How could I do that? I could not afford to eat at restaurants they dined in at. I could not afford to live where they lived. I could not go to the places they went to because I was not at their level. Suddenly, an idea came to me. I thought about it, I did not know how to become successful, but I thought about my mentor John he helped me to get out of my house. I just needed to find someone to help me, so I went for a walk thinking about of finding a solution for this idea. Immediately I saw a carwash. I passed this carwash almost every day walking to go to work, "how did this idea never came to my mind?" I thought. I saw expensive cars going there to be cleaned I remember sometimes I stay there for couple minutes to observe the cars and dream of having a luxury car one day. So, I thought, If I worked there, I would be around rich and successful people! Eventually, I would be able to convince one of them to teach me how to become successful, or a lease I will be motivated to see other people already have what I wanted to have. So that day I decided to start working there. I shared with my friends the idea of leaving landscaping where I made seven dollars an hour to make three dollars plus tips. Everyone told me I was crazy, how are you going to survive with this salary. I thought about it for a second, but then I realized the only reason why I was there was because I allowed other people to make my decisions. I was not willing to let anyone to influence my life again. Only the persistent are the ones who will reach to the top. I said, "I would quit landscaping and get a job washing car." My friends at the job laughed at me. They said, "You cannot speak English. How are you going to communicate with them to ask for help?" I realized they were right, but I did not allow their opinion to decide my future. I did not pay attention to their comments because they were the same as me, why I should pay attention to someone that has not achieved anything in life, I thought. So, if English was a problem, I had to start teaching myself English. Since I cannot afford to pay for classes I took advantage of the people around me. Whenever I was around anyone that could speak English, I would point to objects and ask for the word in English. It was very uncomfortable, but I forced myself to do it. Every day after work, I spent hours and hours learning English. I would read street signs, license plates, and books. I did whatever I could, so I could learn English. Everyone had their own way to learn, and I had mine. In this moment, I was determined to learn English. I knew once I could communicate my life would change. I would spend hours, days, weeks and months teaching myself English. There were many cases people had to ask me to repeat what I was saying because of my heavy accent. There were moments where I felt uncomfortable and wanted to give up. I was not willing to live in the past, not even in my future, because my future demonstrated that I never received what I expected. The only thing I had was the present and only what I did now would determine my future.

Within a few months, I spoke enough English to have a decent conversation. I had a very heavy accent, but I was no longer afraid to speak. Instead of seeing my accent as a weakness, I realized it was a strength. Even though I was not born in America and not able to speak perfect English, I would not use that as an excuse to prevent me from reaching my goals. I woke up, and I was finally back on track for the first time in years, I began to feel hope. I was willing to face my fears and my obstacles. I had a good reason to do it and if your reason is significant enough you find the courage to face any obstacles.

I quit my job working in landscaping and went to work at the carwash. I made less money, but had that dream again, that hope burning in my gut. I realized to move forward; I had to take a step back. What looked like a stupid move to others, would turn out to be the decision that led to my success. I worked hard and did the best job I knew how with every car I cleaned. I kept my eyes open for the right person to approach that would help me to realize my dreams. I still had a great deal of doubt. Why would a successful person want to take the time and extra work to help me? As a child, my mother used to always say, "If a rich person approaches you, it means they want something. If you don't have anything to offer, they won't waste their time". I was about to learn if this was true. I wanted to prove it to myself, I won't believe in anyone who told me is not possible, I am going against to my principles, to my own belief because I know if I want a change in my life I need to change. I thought, "there's nothing to lose and everything to gain. Why should I worry?" I knew this was the only opportunity to be able to achieve my dreams. I couldn't screw up this time. I practiced every day in front of the mirror what I would ask when I found the right person to become my mentor. I looked at myself in the mirror; I looked at every single detail of my face, my hand gestures, and how I would approach this person once I had him in front of me. I dreamed of it and imagined every scenario possible. I did everything I had to do to prepare for that moment. I thought I was going crazy; I was obsessed with becoming successful. I stopped going out with friends, visiting my usual hangouts, and I stopped watching Television. Instead, I dedicated all my time to learning English and planning my new life. I said all I needed was the opportunity to find someone who is willing to help me. As a poor man the only thing I had was my desires and motivation, these two things helped me to keep going, to stand up, to make the difference. I wanted to be rich and I wanted to retire young. How can I retire rich and young when I was living paycheck to paycheck?

There is always someone out there that will help you to achieve your goals. You must get out of your comfort zone and approach them to ask for help. Many people may say no, but if you keep trying, one day that one person that says yes will dramatically change your life for the better. As I said earlier it takes one phone call, one visit to the doctor, one letter or your boss to call you to the office to turn your life upside down, but it can also take you one action, one question, one person to change your life for good. Do not wait any longer to look for this person who is going to transform your life, if you think you deserve more than what you have then get out of your comfort zone and find someone who will help you to achieve your goals. The only reason why you are here now is because you are trained to be here unless you received training in how to be able to go one more step, you won't be able to see it.

After a couple of months working at the carwash, I found him. But before I could take advantage of it, fear overcame me. I made too many excuses. My English was not good enough, even though I was getting better every day. I wasn't confident enough to have a conversation that would convince someone to help me. I remembered all my difficulties since I came to America over the past five years. I was afraid to approach anyone to ask for help. I thought they'd see me as other people did in the restaurant – a poor, dirty lowlife. Rejection terrified me. Even with my insecurities, I was alert. I was looking for the right person to come in my life. I had a gut feeling he or she will be there at the car wash. I finally found someone that I believed would help me achieve my goals. He was a regular customer that came in every Sunday driving a beautiful red Ferrari. I made sure to pay close attention to his car and to detail it to perfection, so he would always ask for me. I talked with him for a few seconds each Sunday to make sure he remembered me, but he was reserved. We'd talk, but he'd respond only with yes or no. It was more difficult than I thought, but I didn't let it get me down. I knew my life would change if I could just get him to open up and see me as more than the guy who washes his car. I thought about different strategies to start a deeper conversation with him, but it seemed like nothing worked. He was dry and gave short answers. I talked about my family, and often I'd shared with him some of my dreams and my desires. His reactions made me afraid to ask him for help, but I didn't want to miss the only opportunity to get out of the life that I was living. I wanted to live in a house with my family. I did not want to continue living with other people. By this time my second daughter, Penelope had already been born, so I had to do it not only for me but my entire family. I wanted to take my wife away from working two jobs to support my dream. I wanted to have a car, house and I did not want to worry about my paycheck. I wanted to live in a nice neighborhood where my children could go to good schools and get a great education. I wanted to earn more money. I firmly believed that I deserved more.

Here again, I had to overcome my fears. What do you do when you have the opportunity to change your life for the better? I believe everyone knows somehow what that one thing is not allowing them to take the next step. We all know how to get our dreams to come true, we're just not willing to face the fear and take the next step. That one step you take every day, the closer you are to reach your goal. Eventually, I thought to myself, "What's the worst that could happen? He could complain, and I could lose my job. I work in a carwash. I could easily get another job. The worst he could do is say no." I didn't have much to lose, but I had everything to gain. I had to push through the fear. Every memory of rejection, scorn, discrimination, and pain I had encountered in the past, I had to leave behind. I had to step up, take ownership of where I was in life, and realize that up to this point, it was my fault that I was not a success. I could not blame anyone else. I had to forgive myself for my conformity - for being comfortable with life; for five years of inaction and wasted time; for all my poor decisions and failures. I had made many sacrifices at this point, and I felt this was the only chance that I had. I found the courage to leave the past behind, focus on my present, and embrace my future. I thought to myself that I had to do something before I lost the opportunity. Nervous and uncomfortable, I approached him to ask a question that would drastically change the direction of my life. His influence and the concepts he shared with me drastically changed my life overnight.

The only way that you will receive what you want in life is if you are unwilling to allow the rejection, the judgment, your surroundings and your vulnerability to take over your life. You need to wake up and take charge NOW. Sometimes we are one question away, one decision away, or one fear that we need to face away. What are you waiting for?

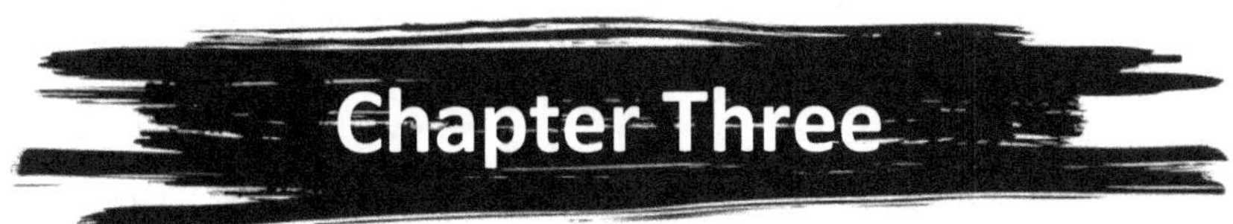

Chapter Three

Don't Be Afraid to Ask for Help

That Sunday morning in August 2006, I decided to approach him, to face my fears and to overcome my obstacles. For months, I had searched for someone to teach me how to overcome my obstacles by asking a simple question. There is always someone willing to share their knowledge and I was destined to find that person. For some time, I thought this person was here at the car wash. I did not know anyone before, but I just had a gut feeling; I want to ask how do I become successful?

It was a crazy idea, but the only solution I had. I was living paycheck to paycheck and had no savings. I was sharing a house with several other people. I still had terrible behaviors I learned not only from childhood but throughout my life. I had been preparing myself for this moment. I had practiced what I would say to him for months. I stood in front of the mirror and practiced how I would ask the most important question of my life. It took many weeks because I knew I had to get this right. I could not afford to fail one more time. I was tired of failing. I was desperate to learn how to become someone different. I identified my choice and created the opportunity that would help to change my life.

I approached him Sunday and I said, "Steve, can I ask you a question?" He said, "Sure Manny. What's up?" I was prepared to ask the question, but I froze! I was so nervous, I couldn't even speak! My entire future, the future of my family, depended on his answer. The magnitude of that moment overwhelmed me, and I could not get the words out. He stood there waiting and waiting, but I couldn't do It. I couldn't get the words out. I said, "Never mind. I will tell you next time." This happened for a couple of weeks. So much was riding on his answer that I had to overcome my fear of his rejection and ask him the question that would help to change my life. I thought to myself once again, "What do I have to lose? I crossed the ocean and uprooted myself and my family to pursue my dream; I left a comfortable situation to live the most uncomfortable life I could ever imagine. So far in my life I have dropped the seminar, I dropped of college, I almost lost my life with my first wife, I left my family behind, I ate out of a trash can; I walked for miles in the cold winter in New Jersey without a jacket. I had been through so many difficult situations. Now standing in front of me was the only opportunity I had to affect the change I wanted, so I had to take advantage of it. The worst that could happen was for him to say no and complain to the manager. I could lose my job, but I work in a carwash. I had lost so many things at this point that losing a dead-end job would not be so bad. I could easily replace this job. With that thought in mind, I finally gained the courage to approach him.

Here it was, another Sunday. As I finished detailing the Ferrari, with a gut full of courage, I approached him again. I said, "Steve, I have been trying to ask you a question for the last couple weeks, but I am not sure how to ask you. I was nervous, my hands and my legs were shaking. But I continue talking, to tell the truth, I really want you to help me to become successful. I love the way you dress… the car you drive, the clothes you wear. I want to accomplish those things for myself. I came to America with big dreams and ended up in a worse place than I ever thought my life could be. This is not me, I'm ambitious and long for a better life. I've been trying for the last five years and I cannot find the way to be successful. I am the first immigrant from my family in America; I don't know anyone here that can help me and teach me the way to overcome my fears and to be rich like you. Can you please teach me how to be as successful as you are?" The relief. Finally, I got it out. However, he didn't answer. He just looked at me. He stared into my eyes. It felt like forever, but was probably only about thirty seconds, the longest thirty seconds of my life. He was sizing me up, trying to see how sincere I was. A lot of things crossed my mind, the nervousness did not allow me to think positive. I was afraid he would say "no" but at the same time I was hoping everything came out well for the first time in a long time. What can you expect when you have many things that go wrong in your life. I wanted to give myself another opportunity to believe in myself and believe in the good intention of other people. I knew he was the right person for this reason, but what he did next surprised me. He put his hand in his pocket, pulled out a business card and handed it to me. He said, "Manny meet me at my office tomorrow morning at 8 am."

"One of the greatest discoveries a man makes, one of his great surprises, is to find he can do what he was afraid he couldn't do. I have learned over the years that when one's mind is made up, this diminishes fear; knowing what must be done does away with your concern."

I can't describe how excited I was. I knew without a doubt that after that day my life would be different. I did not know how I would achieve it, but I knew he would help me to get there. Finally, I was realizing my dream. No more mindless labor. I was no longer a faceless person. I would work hard and learn all I needed to become successful. I was amazed. I realized my life had just changed because I was not afraid to ask for help. Steve, my new mentor, said "YES." I immediately called all my friends who made fun of me, who said no one would help me to achieve success. I was ready to prove that when you follow your dreams, visualize the life that you want to live, and you prepare yourself for the opportunity a miracle is bound to happen in your life.

That day was one of the most fantastic days of my life. I knew it would be a game changer for my entire family. Our lives would be changing drastically. The days of been longer a common laborer washing cars was almost about to end. I did not have to worry about my future, I will be focus in building my present, my new life and I was ready to transform my life around. I knew lot of changes will be happening to me. I can't describe to you the joy and excitement I felt. I felt like a new man, just the fact he was willing to help me, changed my perspective, I saw possibilities in my life, there was hope and a way to succeed. At that moment, a new door opened for me, and I was ready to jump through it. A whole new life was in front of me. That new life had always been there. I just did not know how to access it until I made the decision to change my life, to ask for help. I turned around my actual circumstances by taking accountability instead of blaming everyone else. I took a chance, faced my fears and asked for help. I did not know what he was going to teach me, but what I did know was this man was rich and successful, and he was willing to teach me how I could become that too. There always will be others that are willing to help you as long you genuinely ask. He had seen me in the car wash for months. He knew I was struggling in life, but he never offered to help me until I decided to approach him and ask for help. Sometimes I think about my life, how I would be if I did not take the courage to ask for help. I can tell you, I probably will be doing the same type of job, making a minimum wage. I was on the way to make a legacy for my descendants.

I went back to Lakewood, New Jersey not long ago to visit the town to look for people that I knew. I went to different places I worked at, to my surprise I found many people with whom I shared the same house, or we usually worked together, some were still working landscaping, others were working at the car wash and others where working in factories. What happened with them? Why are they still doing the same type of job? Living the same life, hanging out with the same type of friends. The only valid reason why is because they are not willing to face their fears. Unless you are willing to face your fears, you will be doing the same job living your same mediocre life.

"Be not afraid of discomfort. If you're unable to put yourself in a situation where you're uncomfortable, then you will never grow. You will never change. You will never learn. If you're not able to tolerate a little pain and discomfort, you will never be better."

As I left the carwash that day, I rode the bus home and smiled the whole time staring at his business card. I was envisioning how my life would change. I thought about my difficulties since I came to America. Finally, after five years, I was on the way to regaining my life, my dreams, and my possibilities again. I paid the price. I made all the sacrifices and lost many battles.

The next morning, I woke up early. I didn't want to miss a second of my new life. I felt like a kid with a new toy. He asked me to be there at 8 am; I was there at 6 am. I was so surprised that when I arrived at his office two hours early, he was already there. He immediately had me come into his office and said, "I was not expecting you to be here so early." I replied, "I want to show you how much this means to me and how badly I want to be successful." He said, "I will give you one hour every Monday for the next six months, and I'll teach you everything that I know. Today, since you came early, I will give you two hours." He was generous, caring, but I was nervous. Steve had a beautiful office in an exclusive area. Everything from the desk to the pictures on the wall were spectacular. The view of the city from his office amazed me. I spent the first hour telling him my story. He was captured by it and felt humbled to meet someone like me. He said, "Manny, the tactics I am about to teach you, no one will learn in college. It is not in books, and the people who know about it will never share it with others. I want to say that I have been visiting the carwash for years and nobody ever dared to approach me, except for you." At that moment, I knew I had done the right thing. He made me feel special, comfortable allowing me to open and share my desires.

"The first lesson I want to teach you today you already know." I thought to myself, "I knew it!" He said, "Successful people are not afraid to ask for help. They understand they do not have to know everything. Successful people understand they have strengths, but they also know they have tons of weaknesses. Let me say if you want to reach a goal, but you don't know how to achieve it, you probably do not have all the resources you need. Successful people find someone that has already achieved what they want to achieve. They will help you get there or point you in the right direction. The bottom line is, if you want to reach your goals, you must move out of your comfort zone. You must be uncomfortable to be comfortable. Successful people keep it moving and always adapt to any situation. They learn from their own experiences and the experiences of others. They read constantly; they look for ways to improve themselves every day; to be better than they were the day before." I thought about everything he told me. I had to ask, "How do I know if I'm moving out of my comfort zone?" I also asked for suggestions in books.

He said, "Any time you are doing something that you really don't want to do, or if it makes you feel uncomfortable, scared, or you lack confidence, is when you know you are moving out of your comfort zone. Even more important, you know you're growing. If you move out your comfort zone, you grow. But if you stay still doing the same thing, you will never achieve anything."

"You have to have a clear understanding of what you want in life. It's like driving a car without a destination. You'll be surprised how many people never achieve their goals because they're afraid to ask for help or they don't know what they really want, where they're going and how to get there."

There are always opportunities to learn and grow, to be better than ourselves and to outshine our expectations. You don't have to have every answer, and you don't have to know how everything is done. But you benefit when you know where to go for help when you're in need, and then to avail ourselves of those resources. You must look for people that can help you to learn new skill. In business, it's more important with who you know than what you know.

I wanted to learn more. I wanted to take this opportunity to learn as much as possible. Right then, I knew I was in front of someone wise, someone willing to teach me - not just simple techniques and beliefs, but powerful steps to radically change my life. It was my responsibility to become engaged, to become active in pursuit of a complete change, a complete overhaul. It wouldn't be easy, but I was willing to pay the price and work harder than ever. I asked, "What can I gain by asking for help?" He replied. There are many benefits to asking for help. It all depends on your actual circumstances, but I want to share a few.

"Success is never an accident. Your positive actions combined with positive thinking, results in success. Success is the result of hard work, learning from failure, pushing past your comfort zone and persisting in the face of fear. Put your heart, mind, and soul into even your smallest acts and you will succeed."

Move forward

It will help you to move out of your comfort zone It will give you the opportunity to do something different to get "unstuck," and learn how to proceed in any situation. It will prepare you for the future.

The person that you ask for help should have already achieved what you are looking to gain. They should already know the road to success.

Can you remember a moment when you hesitated when trying to reach out to someone? Chances are you've felt a certain degree of stress. You may have been concerned until you asked for help, and then felt the relief of gaining the answers you needed. The forward momentum also means growing. Your life will not be stagnant, and you will be closer to achieving your goals.

I could not imagine my life without others. I thought about my first mentor, the priest. He came into my life at the moment I needed a father figure, a critical age. Looking back, he was the best thing that could have happened to me. He protected me from making the mistakes most of my friends at the time were making. He changed my life in the right direction. He showed me hope, made me aware of talents and abilities within myself I hadn't discovered. Now, I was in front of someone who steered my life in a completely different direction. I understood the importance of building relationships and I didn't have to do everything myself. Finally, it was clear: I could ask for help. I could ask for support, and I could learn from the wisdom of others. Think about how many times you have lost the opportunity to have something, to get a discount in one product, to get a loan to purchase a car, or simply ask for a favor to save time and money. All these are not allowing you to move forward, they hold you back. What is not helping you to move forward, is pushing you to move forward.

Collaborate

Think about how two or more people can achieve the expected results faster than one person alone. Together we are stronger. Most of the time, we don't ask for help, or feedback Most often, we don't use the experiences of others to help us. We tend to believe if we're not doing the task ourselves it won't be done correctly. We don't want to collaborate. We don't even try. In this millennium, people team up more than ever. Famous people, especially singers, understand the power of a duo or the power of the group or the band. It's why they need others to participate - because your strength could be my weakness. This is a concept we will cover later in greater detail.

I learned feedback is a gift you must humbly receive. When someone provides you with feedback, take it. Whether you like what they have to say or not, you can always learn something from it. The reason someone shares their feedback with you is to make you better; they want the best for you. Asking for feedback will only make you better. Also, you can collaborate with someone by volunteering to partner with someone to complete a job. It will make you feel good because you are helping, but also make the other person feel great because they know they can count on you. This is a great way to build stronger relationships, plus you probably will be discovering skills you never thought you had.

I said, "So you're telling me that tomorrow when I get to the carwash to look for ways to help my co-workers or someone who is struggling with their responsibilities?" "Yes, Manny" he responds. "Once you start doing that, you set yourself apart from everyone else. Then, he asked me questions, "who in your team is looking for ways to help others? Without hesitation, I responded, "no one does that", everyone is looking to do the own thing and then go home. He said, this is the difference between a successful person and an unsuccessful person. Think about how you will be more valuable."

Everyone is out for themselves. They live in their own worlds, and they don't care about others. Your responsibility is to do the opposite, and it will make you a different person. This is the power of discomfort. Not only should you do the opposite of what you want to do, but also do the opposite of what others do." I asked, "What is the power of discomfort?" "The power of discomfort is a technique not many people know about. It is simple to execute, but at the same time very powerful. You must go against your first instinct. Basically, you go against yourself." Let's say you wake up every morning at 7 am to go to work. Moving forward, set your alarm for 6 am to make yourself uncomfortable. Alternatively, you spend four hours a day watching television; moving forward, only watch for two hours. If you hate to read, you should make yourself read for one hour each day. If you love eating fast food, you should only eat it once per week. You do not like to exercise, join the gym or go for a walk or run every day. If you do exercise for 30 minutes, force yourself to do 45 minutes. If you like to drink soda, every time you want to drink soda you will choose water. It doesn't matter; whatever your habits are now, you can change them. Leaders understand they need to go against their habits. By going against yourself, you are growing, a will place you in the front row. You will be doing what others are not willing to do it. I said, "I always was willing to do what others did not want to do. I always worked in a job others did not want to work." He smiles and replied. "Manny, one thing is to do the job no one wants to do, and the other thing is to be willing to do things others do for comfort, things that challenge yourself, things that make you better, things that help you grow.

Leaders understand the power of discomfort. Leaders hate to be comfortable. They know the brain is always looking to make you happy and comfortable. They go against their first instinct to gain control over their lives, over their being. The power of discomfort makes you show up for a meeting one hour before the meeting starts; dial into a conference call 10 minutes before the call starts; allow others to participate first before they express their point of view; they are always well prepared before any event or task. People think that successful people make good decisions every day. In reality, they make a few great decisions and manage them well. You can make good decisions every day, but if you do not learn how to manage them, you won't go very far. For that reason, it is essential that you start by managing yourself first before you pretend to manage others."

I'm going to prove it to you. He asked me. "Have you ever made a New Year's resolution?" I said, "Yes, every year." He asked me, "How many of the New Year's resolutions have you accomplished?" I said, "None. I always stopped after my first couple of months." He smiled. "That is my point. People focus more on making decisions than managing the decisions. So, the result becomes a lack of commitment, discipline, purpose, and engagement. Besides, most people do not stick to their commitment. They give up after the first try. They expect things to happen quickly. When you commit to something, stick with it until it is done. Do not give up. Look for help and ask for feedback and you will find a way to succeed. It is uncomfortable, but it is the only way."

As the weeks pasted, I was impressed with the lesson I was receiving. I imagined how my life would be. For the first time, I would learn concepts no one had ever taught me before. He was the right person for me. It's simple: Find the right person, and it makes a considerable difference. It is fundamental to achieving any level of success. I thought, "What would I have missed if I didn't dare to ask for help." I could feel my excitement growing; It was like a dream come true. In every meeting I was taking notes. I did not want to miss any detail. I wanted to be able to practice everything until I became an expert.

Achieve your goals in less time

"You must constantly look for people that can help you to achieve your goals. You will save valuable time. Instead of trying to figure out how to do a task, others will guide you and show you the way. Also, as I mentioned before, everything works both ways. You'll find people that can help you, but you also need to look for these people that need your help. The magic of having goals is once you write them down and begin acting on them, you will find people that are willing to help you. Some may ask if you need help, while others you have to take the initiative to approach and ask for help, the same as you did Manny."

Time is valuable: We all have 24 hours to achieve our daily goals. The only difference is successful people utilize their time wisely, while others don't. I asked, how do I know the importance of time and how I can be more productive with my time? He replied. "There are many ways to do it, also there is a way on how to plan your day more effectively, but now I want to give an example to help you to understand the value of time." I was so excited to hear about how I could manage my time better and what I should do to make more time to do the things that will take me closer to my goal. He asked me how old I was. I said "26." He replied. The average American dies at 78 if they die of natural causes. Do the math for me, if you are 26 and you die at the age of 78 how many years left do you have to leave." I said, "52." Now multiply for 365 days. I said 18,980 days. Then he stopped talking and let digest this information. As I was looking at the number of days I had left, it did not feel much. In some ways he made me see that I did not have much time, even though I was young it didn't feel like much.

Then he said there is one way you can gain time. Most successful people apply this to their lives. He asked me at what time I woke up every day? I replied. "I wake up at 7 am. "He said. I am going to teach you how you can live for an additional four years until you died." At first, I was skeptical; I did not understand, what does the time I wake up have to do with living four additional years? He said, "successful people wake up at five, and some at four am every morning. By you waking up two hours before the time you are waking up now, you will be gaining two additional hours every day, 730 hours per year, in your 52 years left represent 4.33 years. People pay millions of dollars to have one additional day in their life. Think about it."

Learn new skills

"You will be learning new skills; you will be learning from the experiences of others; from their mistakes. How great would life be if we could avoid most of our mistakes by connecting with those leaders that have already walked your same path? I have learned not to make any important decisions without seeking the opinion of others. I have avoided many mistakes that would end up costing me millions of dollars. Now it is essential to ask the right person. Don't do what the 95% of people do." "What is that?" I asked. He replied, "They ask a friend, family member, or coworker for their opinion. If you look at their background, they have not achieved any level of success. You do not go to a plumber to fix your teeth or go to the police for advice on accounting. You must know if this person has been successful in the area that you need. You want to be rich. That's why you came to me. I can only teach you what I know. If I gave an opinion about something that is not my expertise, I probably wouldn't give you the right answer."

Thinking about how many times we've had great ideas, but we make the terrible mistake of asking someone who doesn't know anything about the topic and even worse someone that have never achieved any level of success. It happened to me many times, I asked the wrong person for opinion, for advice. At that moment I was thankful I did not pay attention to my peers when I was seeking their opinion when I was going to apply to work at the car wash. This life lesson was an eye-opener for me, change the perspective of my life. I am sure you probably think about how many times this has happened to you, that you came excited to share a great idea with a friend or anyone you know, and they told you it was a not a good idea, but, they have never achieved anything important in their life.

Gain new Strengths

"You will discover talents and abilities that never believed yourself to have. You will be able to discover your potential, and most important, you will learn more about yourself than ever before. People think that asking for help is a weakness. In fact, it is a strength that once mastered, your life will change drastically. Understanding your abilities will help you gain confidence. It is easier to gain confidence when you are learning from someone that has already faced the same situation and succeed, they can guide you on the best path to follow. I am not saying you will always find the easy way to do things in life. I want to make sure that you understand there is no easy way to achieve success, but with the guidance of others, you will be able to find success too. While others spend the rest of their lives trying to figure things out and trying to overcome their weakness, others understand the power of discomfort. They are not comfortable with what they have already achieved; they continually look for ways to improve the strategies and master their strengths. If you surround yourself with these types of people, they will influence you just by being around them."

Learning goes both ways

"When you collaborate, you not only learn from others, but they also learn from you. Think about someone that comes to you for help; both of you will grow. They will learn from you, and you will learn from the experience."

Looking through my notes and thinking about these lessons, I was glad I made the right decision. For the first time, I went to the right person to learn about the power of discomfort. As time passed and the conversation grew deeper, my interest in learning about this concept was growing. I felt so excited about my new direction in life; about my new mentor, and most important, the lessons I was offered. I saw the possibilities; I felt hope and inspiration. Just to be around someone that had achieved such great success in a short period of time was a terrific experience for me.

Asking for help doesn't devalue you. It can enable you to advance and connect you meaningfully with others, bolster your productivity and ability to do things with greater ease, and better prepare you for your next challenge in life.

He was teaching me the right thing. How many times do we have access to people we know are successful, yet we passed up that opportunity to ask for help or advice? Ask to collaborate with them on a project or activity. As he was talking about the importance of asking for help and finding a mentor, I thought back on my entire life. How through my ignorance - or arrogance - I passed up several opportunities. The conversation was an eye-opener for me. It changed my perspective on life, and how do I saw myself and others.

As I reflected on our conversation, I remembered he said "There is nothing worse than fear. It paralyzes you and does not allow you to grow. Fear is a lack of confidence. You gain confidence by practicing and practicing until you feel good about yourself doing the task. If I place you in front of a camera on a television show without any rehearsal, you will probably freeze, not say anything, or say a lot of things that don't make sense. You would be terrified. On the other hand, if you had been doing television for five years in your country and now you come to America, and I give you the same opportunity, you would probably do well and easily succeed. Once you are confident, the fear disappears, but you also need to be willing to pay the price. Be uncomfortable, get feedback, practice and become better than yourself every day if you want to be successful. Eagles fly. Chickens don't."

Look at your past. Do you know of a person that if you dared to ask for help and they agreed, your life would have changed? If your answer is yes, what are you waiting for? Take action! Get out of the comfort zone. I know that you want to move to the next level; you want to move one step up; you want to continue moving forward. If you can't think of someone, then you must actively look for the person that can help you to move to the next level. There are other people like you reading this book and taking action now, thinking about their strengths, thinking about who they want to ask for help. If you believe like me in the power of discomfort you must understand fear does not allow you to be you, to explore your full potential.

As I look back on my life, I do not know where I would be at this moment if I did not ask for help. As you grow in your career or your business, you become an expert. You will relate with people that have a different mentality, different mindset, and a different perspective on life. Your life will change drastically. I have used this concept of asking for help since then. Some people call them mentors, others call them friends. But they are simply someone who has changed the course of your life. Everyone has a least one person who has changed their life. It could be someone that sees something in you that you did not see in yourself or someone who gave you your first opportunity. Even when you did not believe in yourself, they believed in you. It could be a teacher, a family member, a friend that inspired you, or a boss who discovered the talent and abilities in you.

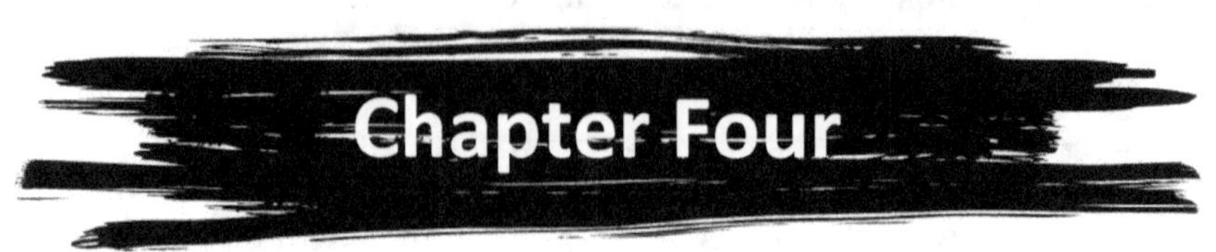

Develop Your Leadership Style

During our weekly meetings, I asked Steve another question. "My dream is to become a leader. I want to be able to lead others, but I have no one to lead. I am not even sure if I have the skills, but I understand to be successful in life I need to have a strong foundation on the basis of leadership. Can you teach me different leadership styles and what I need to know about managing people?"

He responded: "If you want to be a great leader, begin by leading yourself. If you can't lead your thoughts, your emotions; if you can't manage your time, your commitments, your goals, your priorities, your life, your surroundings, your behaviors/gestures, and your words, no one will follow you. Leaders have one thing clear; they understand their actions speak louder than their words. For this reason, they do not have to say a lot for others to follow. Others will recognize you once you achieve this position. You will start leading by example. They have something in common; they sit, talk, walk, act, think the same way. You must learn how to manage yourself daily and consistently. They understand that others constantly observe them. They know of their behaviors and surroundings. They master the power of discomfort."

"I know this is a lot of information, but I want to break it down for you," he said. "I want to divide this into three categories, Body Language, Manage your Intonation, Manage your Words."

"When you meet someone for the first time, they have five seconds to form an impression of you. They observe the way you are dressed, the way you walk, talk, sit, even how you use your computer or your cell phone."

At that moment I knew I had to make changes in my life inside and outside. He looks at me for a few minutes, I felt uncomfortable at first but later I understand he wanted to send me a message that if I want to be a leader, or someone others will follow I need to change my appearance.

Body Language

As leaders, we need to understand how to manage our gestures. Using our hands, our face, our body positioning, eye contact, and how we dress. You must sell yourself to others 24/7. Some people take advantage of this, and others don't. However, a great leader understands this is over 59% of his leadership. For that reason, they pay close attention to their behaviors. You need to use specific gestures in your conversation. He stood up and taught me several gestures and when to use them. I asked, "How do I practice these gestures if I have no one to lead?" He replied, "I recommend you practice while you are on the phone speaking with anyone. Go to the mall to volunteer yourself to help people or give directions to others. When you want a coffee with sugar, don't just say three sugars; use the gestures. When you go to the gas station, practice with the people there. They do not know you; they won't criticize or judge you. I call them a neutral audience. It is the best place to practice your leadership skills. The habit makes the monk."

Manage Your Intonation

"Managing your tone of voice is critical. It is 38% of communication. Have you ever heard the phrase, 'It is not what you say, but how you say it? 'Using the proper intonation combined with your body language is vital in leading. Intonation is the pitch pattern of your voice. It conveys meaning because your voice must convey meaning. If you speak in the same tone, don't emphasize essential words and your message has no passion or believability, your point won't be clear, and you won't be able to lead."

He taught me different exercises to practice. They were simple, but powerful. He recommended I practice daily: on the way to work or on my way home– "any time you are alone, practice," he said. Your tone of voice will change, and others will follow you more because your voice will convey sincerity and trustworthiness.

He also made me watch a few videos. One from Dr. Martin Luther King Jr. and another from John F. Kennedy. He said the power of their speech was not the message, but how they conveyed it, how they delivered it. The way you speak with others is essential — and you must master it. Great leaders know when to express emotion and when to hold it back. Managing your intonation is uncomfortable, but once you practice and master it, your leadership will improve. Based on your intonation, people will decide if they want to continue listening to you or not. In other words, intonation refers to the rise and fall of pitch and tone when speaking, which stresses relevant words to make your speech more exciting and compelling. Without intonation, your voice will be flat like a robot's. You won't have flavor and you'll be uninteresting It must be a combination of pitch, pace, power, and tone. He spent significant time explaining how to become a better communicator over the next few weeks.

His exercises made me walk and talk differently. My friends immediately noticed a change in my demeanor. My coworkers noticed, and I noticed myself. I felt like I could do more. I was doing a good job leading and managing myself. I was walking and speaking differently. I went to the mall to practice, in the grocery store, anywhere. In the beginning, I was uncomfortable, but once I overcame my fears, it was easier. For years I wanted to be successful, to stop washing cars, to give myself the courage to do it and forced myself to be uncomfortable.

Increase Your Value

Do you know someone you feel adds value to your life? Think of how much you respect them. Adding value to others is one of the most critical skills for a leader. When you add value, you can change a person's life. You can help them uncover talents and abilities they were unaware of. I have known many people throughout my life that have changed me in so many positive ways. The importance of adding value to others is reflected in how much they learn from you and in return, how much you learn from them in the process. You also get to practice and become better in any area. People are paid based on the value they add to their employer. The more you have to offer, the more you learn and diversify your skills, the more money you can make. Personally I dedicated 1% of my salary to buying books. Mostly audiobooks in the beginning as my English was still improving and I utilized my travel to listen and further my skills. This can be as simple as riding in the car to the gym or to the grocery store. Dedicate as least one hour a day to learn something new. Knowledge is power and a well-educated mind can travel distances and discover talents before hidden to them.

People Influence

Have you ever heard the saying, "Show me your company and I will tell you who you are?" Or, "If you lay down with dogs, you get up with fleas?" Many people surround themselves with those who are bad influences. They follow the crowd, make poor decisions and end up as bad as their influences.

I knew a family that had two children. Both were educated the same way, went to the same school, had the same level of education. Both ate the same foods. Their parent treated them the same way, and they grew up in the same environment. When they went to high school, they hung out with different friends. One gravitated toward sports and had friends with those same interests. They were competitive and worked for good grades. They followed the rules, valued their friendships, and were successful in life. The other kid hung out with a different crowd, with kids who liked to party, do drugs, drink, and didn't care about schoolwork and good grades. Clearly, the first child ended up being successful, with a fantastic career, a stable family and remarkable life. The other child dropped out of high school, got addicted to drugs, became a repeat felon. He never married and became a burden and disappointment to his family. This is a classic example of how you are influenced by the people you surround yourself with. As a leader, it's vital you spend time with people that will make a positive impact in your life.

To illustrate this, Steve gave me a piece of paper and asked me to write my significant goal in life. He then told me to write my five best friends, the people I spent the most time with. He had me write what each one of them did for a living. What I discovered opened my eyes. At the end of this exercise, I realized none of my friends had anything to do with my primary goal. I had not surrounded myself with others that would help influence me towards achieving my goals. Another way to complete the exercise is to write the salary of your top five closest friends, including yourself. If you are at the top of the list, it is a sign you must adjust your friendships. If you are the best in your circle of influence, it is time for you to change your friends. This sounds a little harsh, I must admit, but it is the best way to make the necessary changes in your life.

His lessons invigorated me and opened my mind to a new way of thinking. Learning about the power of discomfort was changing my life. He also showed me how to apply this concept to little things in my daily life. I immediately changed my behavior. Leaving each day, I would speak with others, say hello, goodbye; I'd wish them a good day. If I had a seat on the bus, I would stand and offer my seat to a woman or a senior. I became conscious of my actions and paid close attention to little things. Slowly, my attitude changed towards others and myself.

Over the following weeks, I applied the tips Steve taught me. It felt great. I woke up and got to work an hour earlier. I helped my coworkers, asked my boss for more responsibility and, most importantly, began building great relationships with others. At work, I was first in and the last out. Everyone noticed my change; I noticed a change; my family and friends noticed a change. I didn't feel miserable anymore. Each evening when I got home, I felt grateful and enjoyed the moments with my family even during difficult circumstances. That is the power of discomfort. I believe you should not wait to act the part and demonstrate the behaviors observed of a leader until you are promoted. Be who you strive to be on a daily bases on you will be noticed for your abilities naturally.

He drastically changed my life. He showed me a different perspective. I was learning from the right person. It gave me another opportunity to live. I was determined to protect my new lifestyle. Becoming uncomfortable to achieve my goals was a mantra I echoed in my mind at every moment. I always used it, with every activity, action, and decision, I applied the principle of discomfort. The power of discomfort gave me the energy necessary to keep up and keep going. When working out and running at the gym, my legs grow tired, and I wanted to stop, but instead I pushed myself to be uncomfortable and run for another 15 minutes. It has provided me with a well of strength, energy, and inspiration to keep going.

Now I understood that I did not have to be afraid of anything, because successful people are not fearful to ask for help or express their points of view. Many of my fears went away; I was not scared of having to talk to people, converse in small groups, or even change the topic in a conversation in small ways. If I wanted to be successful, I needed to act like it, think like it, and surround myself with successful people.

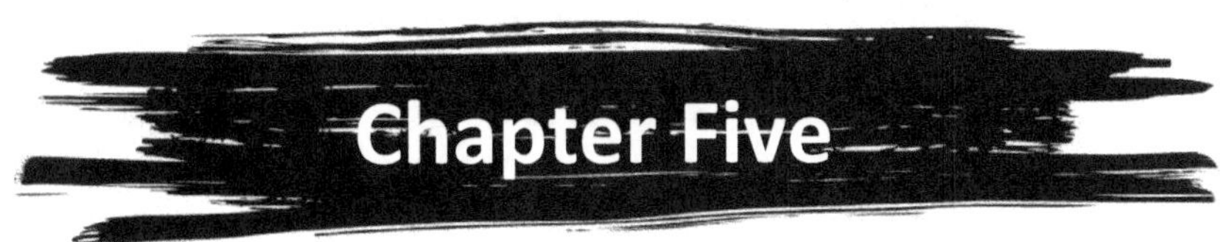

Master Your Strengths

Over the next several weeks, I learned many ways to lead people, and how to lead myself. I also learned about my strengths. I did not understand at first why mastering my strengths was so important until he explained it. As we had our meetings, I realized I was programmed with the wrong chip. Everything I learned in school, from society, and my family, was wrong.

He said: "Before I explain to you the importance of mastering your strengths, I want you to know that your mind has been programmed the wrong way. Unless you change your mindset, you won't be able to win." He was right, think about school. When you are not good in a subject, they force you to study and spend more time on it to get better grades. They train you to focus on your weaknesses. If you are not good at math, they force you to spend a lot more time on the assignments. You stay after class for extra help. You may even have to get a tutor. You end up spending so much time on the subject that is your weakness. If you go to talk to the teacher, they immediately share with you the problems your child has and the ways they can improve, not what they are doing great. Since you were little, you learned that you need to focus on your weakness and not on your strengths.

He asked me to name a singer that I would go to see at a live concert. I mentioned the name. He said, "When you go to a concert, there is a lot that goes into getting everything ready for the fantastic experience. There is someone in charge to book the arena; others set up the sound; the perfect the lighting; they complete the advertising and promotions; others sell the tickets, and some oversee security. The list is long, but before the singer steps on that stage to perform, all these people must do their job. This is what they do best. Now the singer shows up in a limo, gets ready to perform, then goes on stage to sing for an hour. He or she does what they do best, they sing. The singer becomes a master at singing; they only work on their strengths; they hire someone else to take care of the weaknesses. They don't worry about them. They focus on making sure the hour is valuable for everyone by singing to perfection and pleasing the crowd. They practice each day to become better at that one thing they do best."

The way he described it made a great deal of sense. I had spent my life trying to overcome my weaknesses. They are my weaknesses for a reason. With practice, you can get better, but you never will master them. At that moment, I remembered something that happened in the seminary. I wanted to join the choir. Members of the choir could leave every Sunday to sing in the Cathedral. I signed up to join. I practiced with my friends that could sing for months in preparation, but when the time came to audition, the master told me no. I tried for a year to learn how to sing, but singing was my weakness and therefor they did not accepted me into the group.

He then handed me a piece of paper and directed me to write five of my strengths, and five weaknesses. He gave me ten minutes to complete this exercise. It was easy for me to come up with weaknesses; things I felt I needed to improve on. It was extremely difficult to come up with any strength. In those ten minutes, I could not come up with one. I handed the paper back to him with the strengths section blank. Why was it so hard for me to define my strengths? He explained that most people don't know themselves. They have a hard time defining what they are good at, and because of this, they lack direction and focus. It is one reason people don't become successful.

That moment was another huge epiphany for me. I realized most of my life, I had been focusing all my energy in the wrong area. I was so focused on my weaknesses I did not define and improve my strengths. I always thought to become successful I needed to be good at everything; when in reality, I needed to focus on my strengths and become an expert in that area. I needed to find what made me unique, develop in this area and be better at it than most other people. This is where I would become an asset and add value to any employer.

I spent time developing myself in one area. I became better than I was the day before. I continued this every day. I read books on that topic, learned from others, surrounded myself with people that had achieved success in the same area. I followed his advice and if you do the same, I guarantee you will excel and become a master in that area.

Be Patient—Be Consistent

He also said: "Manny, you must be patient to achieve your goals. You must wait for the results. If you are persistent and work at it every day, your day will come." The problem with most people is the lack of patience and consistence. They start a new business, change behaviors, or start a new job, and they are ready to quit after a month because they don't see results. Patience is a virtue that everyone needs to build. If you practice the power of discomfort, you will learn how to exercise patience.

There is a story that tells of three men that attempted a jailbreak. They didn't know how many walls they would have to scale, but they really wanted to escape. They figured there might be only one or two walls, and then they were on their way to freedom. As it turned out, there were several walls they had to overcome. As they climbed the first couple walls, they were energetic and excited.

They knew they were almost home free. They kept going but realized there were more and more walls to scale. They kept climbing, but their excitement faded, and they got tired of doing the work. They couldn't stay focused on the end result of being free. When they reached the ninth wall, they gave up entirely. They turned back. What they didn't realize there were only ten walls. If they had exercised patience and consistency just a little longer, they would have been free.

Thinking back on my life, I realized there were many times I gave up on my dreams. I started projects and never completed them. Instead of being persistent, I gave up and ended right back where I started. Every time you start a new project, change your job, start a new business, basically, we start all over again. I took decades to understand things do not happen quickly. I needed to develop my strengths. I needed to become good at what I'm doing, but I would only achieve all of these if I am consistent and have patience. Most of the time, we are not willing to make the sacrifices, to change our behaviors, to think differently, and to get out of our comfort zone.

As my mentor, Steve, was sharing how he had accomplished many things in his life because of patience, his life lesson helped me to understand the power of consistency. I changed my thinking, redirected my life, and applied the power of discomfort to help me stay focused, practice patience, and applied consistency until I realized success.

Practice Excellence in Your Life

"Manny, the next step on the road of success and to master your strengths, you must excel at what you do." You need to show excellence in all areas of life. Excellence is the quality of being outstanding or performing your task extremely well, the way no one else could do it. To be excellent, you must criticize yourself thoroughly; you must expect the best from yourself and others. If you are going to perform one task, follow the rules. If you are sitting in a meeting, you must be the best in the room. In a family, you must be the best son, daughter, father, mother, brother, sister, uncle, or aunt.

Excellence separates the ordinary from the extraordinary. To be excellent, you must wake up early and work late. You must be curious, self-aware, and take time to think and focus on what is essentially for you. You must be confident, optimistic, help others to achieve their goals. Be humble and create routines that will help you drive the behaviors and the results you expect. Find a mentor and become a mentor to others. Serve others and do unto them as you would want them to do to you.

As the weeks passed, I never missed an appointment with my mentor. I was there every Monday as we agreed. He taught me how to adjust my personal behaviors and how to use discomfort to achieve my goals. I changed my attitude, replaced most of my bad habits, and grew in a way I never thought possible. There was only one problem. Physically, I was still in the same place I was before. I was still washing cars, making the same limited amount of money, and sharing a house with several other people. I was ready and hungry to move to the next stage of my life, to apply his lessons, and jump to my next adventure. I wanted to use my new mindset to achieve success. I didn't know what I would do, but I knew I would not be washing cars for the rest of my life.

As we were talking about excellence and how others will notice you are different when you walk into a room, when you sit in a meeting, when you drive your car, even when you are doing your shopping in the supermarket, he said, "Manny, you must practice excellence in all areas of your life; you don't want to be good in one thing and not good in other things." If you want to be successful, excellence needs to be in your blood. Being excellent is being different. It is doing what others are not willing to do, it is behaving differently than most people. The people who practice excellence in their life have a sense of satisfaction because they know they are doing the right thing. As he was sharing the importance of excellence, I thought about my next move. Steve once said, "When you work for someone, you are helping them to fulfill their dream, not your own." This thought stayed in the back of my mind. It was true. While helping the owner of the car wash fulfill his dream, I was not fulfilling my own. He explained: "It is ok to work for someone, as long as you are working on creating the foundation to make your own dreams become a reality." I knew I wouldn't be there for long, but I was washing the cars like it was my last day on the planet.

During my next meeting with Steve, I shared thoughts about my situation. "Steve," I said, "I have been coming here for a couple of months. I have changed my life in many ways, I have been practicing all the life lessons you have shared with me, but there is one problem. I am still washing cars. I feel I am ready for something bigger. You told me when I am working for someone, I am helping them to fulfill their dream. Now is the time to fulfill my dreams. I know you have done so much for me; more than anyone could ever expect. I need your help to build my own business. Can you help me?" Here I was applying one of the first lessons Steve taught me, asking for help. To my surprise, he was waiting for this moment, but he didn't want to be the one who makes this decision. I thought about how many times I lost an opportunity to become better than myself or to have someone help me because I was not willing to take the first step, to get out of my comfort zone and to face my fear of rejection.

He said, "Manny, I think you are ready to fly. You are an eagle." He also said, "I know a good business where you can perform well and help me at the same time. I own seventeen hundred houses and a few apartment buildings. I need someone to find tenants and rent the properties for me. People are constantly moving, and I need to fill the empty apartments and houses." At that moment, I was impressed. I knew he was rich, but I did not have a clue he owned so many properties, nor that he would give me this opportunity.

"How will I rent these houses for you?" I asked: "Manny, I know you will figure it out." He also shared with me that for every house or apartment I rent, I would receive one month of rent in commission.

At first, I thought this was a bad idea, but once he told me what the average rent was for the properties, I realized it was an excellent opportunity, and I decided I would do it. I said, "I would love to do this job, but I don't have a company, and I don't know anyone. How will I find tenants?" He replied, "With all the knowledge you have now, there is no doubt in my mind you will figure it out."

I left that day the proud owner of my very first business. We registered the company, and I was on my way to fulfilling my dream. I was now a business owner, but I did not have a plan or strategy to proceed. I had to figure out a way to reach a large group of people that needed a rental living space. Even though I had been living in the U.S. for five years, I didn't know many people, and I had no idea how I would find so many renters.

On my way home, I kept thinking about the money I could make. If I rented even one house, I would make more money in commission than I would wash cars for an entire month. Thinking about the potential earnings got my creative juices flowing. I kept thinking about how I could solve this problem. I knew I would need to find a solution. My mind was spinning and I was excited and determined to figure out how I would make my first business a success.

Sometimes in life, we need to focus one hundred percent on what we want to accomplish. Our mind, body and desires need to be aligned towards our goal. You must create the opportunity and solve the challenges you are facing right now. If there is a problem, there is a solution.

While walking home, I saw a sign taped to a light pole that displayed a missing dog. The poster was asking people to call if they had any information about the dog, and at the bottom of the sign was the phone number. The number was written several times so that a person could rip off the small piece that had the number printed but leave the rest of the sign. I noticed that several pieces were missing, but there were still slips of paper left with the phone number. This meant people came and picked up the phone number. At that moment, a light bulb went off in my head as the idea took shape in my mind. What about if I took a picture of a beautiful house and made similar posters advertising property for rent and placed my phone number at the bottom, just like the poster for the missing dog? I could place these posters all over the city. They could be illustrated in every laundromat, grocery store, and library. I realized this was the answer I needed to start my new business. Immediately, I put my plan into action. I spent around one hundred dollars printing posters to hang everywhere. The next day, I went to Steve's office to share my strategy with him. He was so happy that I was able to figure it out within 24 hours, and with a smile on his face, he gave all the keys to empty houses.

My phone did not stop ringing. I was showing the property to over 20 people per day, I was renting properties faster than I expected, and just in my first week, I made over ten thousand dollars renting houses! I couldn't believe I went from making two hundred and fifty dollars a week to ten thousand! As time passed, I made more and more money, my weekly income increased, and I became hungry for more money. I realized different avenues to advertise my business and started utilizing newspapers, radio stations and the internet. My success was booming and I felt established.

A few months passed, I was making enough money to move my family into our own home. We no longer had to share a house with a multitude of people we didn't know where they came from. Purchasing our first home was a huge milestone for us at the time. It made me so happy. I could now afford a car, too. We purchased furniture for the house and our kids could sleep in their own rooms for the first time. We could afford to buy nice clothes, and I could take my family out to eat at nice restaurants. It completely changed our lives.

As I grew, my desire of becoming rich and retiring young, motivated me to look for different ways to make more money and create a different avenue to grow my income. I wanted to be wealthy, but I knew if I wanted to be successful, I needed to do more than just renting houses. Steve was thrilled with my performance. He was not losing any money as the houses were rented almost immediately after they had been vacated. He had a lot of confidence in me, and because of this, I came up with another plan to help drive me closer to my goal.

One day, I met him at his office to share my new job proposition. After we spoke for about ten minutes, I said to him, "Steve, I noticed you have a company that collects the rent for you. I am having a problem because most of the tenants I am renting the houses to, are Latinos, and my tenants speak little English, they cannot communicate with the management company. Every time they have an issue in the house, they call me and then I have to call the management company. The company you've hired can't communicate with them effectively. Every day, they call me to translate. I want to propose that I can do this job for you. Instead of paying them $45 per tenant, I will charge you only $35. You will save money, and the tenants will feel comfortable and have no problems communicating." He looked at me, smiled, and said: "You are so smart." He picked up the phone and fired the other company. I walked out of his office that day with my second business. I now had a second avenue of income.

Thinking about this moment of my life, I created the opportunity, plus I was excellent at what I was doing. He didn't give me the business because he would save ten dollars for a property; remember he was a rich man. He knew I transformed my life, drove the business with excellence and I could assume more responsibilities. There were many occasions when he asked me to perform tasks that didn't fit my business, and I did it even before he expected them. During this time, he understood I could handle more responsibility. Opportunities come only when you are ready to handle them.

I had been working with Steve for over eight months, and at this point, I was renting and managing his properties, but I was ready for more. I wanted to continue taking advantage of this opportunity; I wanted to apply everything I had learned from him into my business. So one day, I was thinking about the business and how I could increase the income. I was brainstorming for ideas to increase my revenue. At that moment, my phone rang, and it was Steve calling to tell me I had to call a company to fix a house where the tenant just moved. An idea arose, "why have I never thought of this?" I asked myself.

I noticed every time a tenant moved out, I had to call a company to change the carpet, paint the walls, fix the floors and make any other home improvements necessary in the house. I saw this as another opportunity to generate additional income. This time, I registered the company and hired twenty experienced home improvement workers. I also purchased a couple of work vans and the tools we would need. Once I was ready, I approached my mentor with the proposition. I would refurbish his vacated properties, charging him 20 percent less than the current company, but only if he would recommend me to his friends and all his contacts. He once again agreed to my proposal. Sometimes in life we have to give people the right motivation to help us grow and achieve more than we ever thought possible.

Within a year, I had built an empire. I was making more money than I ever dreamt of. Beside of this company, I started another, designing, selling and installing kitchen cabinets. I was one of the first designing kitchens in 3D. I made so much money I didn't know what to do with it. I bought properties back home in the Dominican Republic and started helping my mother build a house. My goal was to work for ten more years, saving and investing my money, and retire at 40.

My kids were growing up, and my family was growing larger. Our youngest child, Sheana, was recently born. Penelope was now four years old, Maite was eight, and my son, Manuel Jr., was eleven. I bought a house near the beach. My mentor introduced me to the world of real estate investing. Within a few years, I was successfully buying houses, fixing them up, and renting them as an investment. I felt that all the lessons I had learned over the last couple of years, and all the sacrifices I made by being uncomfortable, really worked. It proved that successful people think and act differently from ordinary people.

Six years ago, when the priest came to tell me to leave the country, my job and my family behind, I never imagined that one day I would have the knowledge and money I now had. Life had a stranger surprise and what would happen a couple months later changed my life completely.

I made many friends and built an excellent reputation in the industry. My company was in demand to complete jobs in roofing, siding, floor repair and installation, bathroom remodeling, basement renovation, and home additions. Life was amazing. I could not ask for more. For the first time, I felt I was living the American dream. It all started from not being comfortable with the life I was living, not allowing my circumstances to determine my future, and most importantly, not being afraid to ask for help. Had I not had the courage to ask for help, then I would not have been able to create the success I enjoyed so much. During this time, I felt all the sacrifices paid off, I was no longer upset with myself.

I understand everything I went through in my life was part of the plan. I learned that, sometimes things don't happen the way you want; instead, happens how it should. Practicing excellence and patience has been fundamental to achieving my goals. I constantly teach people to be successful in any area of your life, you need to prepare yourself, make changes and become better than what you were the day before, even the moment before.

Become a Better Version of Yourself

Later, my mentor shared a technique with me that is simple but powerful. Once I learned, this concept helped me to achieve anything in life, I became stronger then I was before. I was able to understand myself more and knew my behaviors and thoughts. We are responsible for our own success and failure; our daily decisions and actions determine our life. If we want to change our life, we must change our mind.

When Steve told me I needed to change my mind, I asked, "how can I change my mind? How can someone change their belief?" I remember something he mentioned in one of our prior conversations. He said: "Our beliefs determine our thoughts, and our thoughts determine our actions. If you want to achieve success, you must change your beliefs."

I know this sounds crazy - it sounded crazy to me, too, back then, but it's so true. We are where we are because of our beliefs. If you want to achieve anything different, you must change, and this starts by believing in yourself, believing that fears only exist in your mind and that you are responsible for creating possibilities. I said, "Steve, I do understand I need to change my beliefs, I know this is fundamental on the road to success, but how can I change it?" He said: "It is easy to do, just become better than yourself every second and every moment."

"How can I become better than myself every moment?" I asked.

"Let's say after you finish a meeting, a conversation with someone, after you closed a deal, after you have been on vacation, after you made a choice, started a new job, you finished your day, ended your workout, basically after every event in your life, I want you to ask yourself two questions."

As he was talking, I was imagining all the possible events in my life I should ask these two questions, but I was thinking about why I should and how these questions will change my life, but one thing I was sure, I trust Steve, he has proven his knowledge, and his life lessons transformed my life already, and I was looking to jump to the next level, and I knew this would help tremendously.

"I want you to challenge yourself and ask two questions every time you complete a task. "

"What did I do well?"

"What can I do better?"

I said, "You are telling me every time I finish a job, I should ask myself these two questions? When I finish a meeting? Before I go to bed?" He said: "Yes, basically every time you complete a task you should take five minutes of your time to think about what you did well and what you can improve." The problem with a majority of the people is they do not take the time to analyze themselves, to look for ways to improve, to become better and won't think about their goals. They are afraid of themselves.

"I want to give you some homework," he said, "and after you complete the homework, you will understand why most people are afraid to criticize themselves, and for that reason, they do not get better in life."

He asked me to go home and record a video of myself, just a ten-minute video. I could talk about any topic, whatever felt comfortable. At first, I thought this was an easy task; I could record a video. But then he asked me to watch myself in the video. He also said: "I guarantee you won't finish watching yourself for ten minutes." He smiled and sent me home.

I recorded the video and played it back, but after one minute, I was dropping it; I couldn't see myself, I felt horrible. I didn't look good on camera, and I did not have the talent to record a video. At this moment, I understood what Steve was telling me, but I didn't know how he knew I would stop the video. Later that week, he said: "we criticize ourselves harder than others do." I then asked myself those two questions in every event in my life and every time after I change a task. I also taught this concept to the people I mentored. When I asked those two questions, I could identify my strengths and weaknesses. The things I could do better or grow stronger, but I just could not identify what I could do better. I would think about how I would do it the next time given the opportunity. With that, you are setting yourself up for success because once you have the same opportunity in front of you, your brain will find the right answer for you. When you identify the things you believe you are doing well, it sends a sense of accomplishment.

I ask my team after every meeting or after I do a one-on-one sessions these two questions. Not just to myself, but to the other person as well. I can tell you I wouldn't have achieved the level of success if Steve did not teach me those two questions.

I recently met someone while I was visiting a restaurant. He is a fantastic employee who has been working for the company for over 30 years. It was his first job and will probably be his last. While speaking with him, he told me how happy he was in his current position. He knows how to do everything; the job had become so easy to do. He was comfortable. He also mentioned the manager had offered him a better position on many occasions, but he never took the chance to learn something new. Later in the conversation, I asked a couple of other questions. He mentioned he has always been afraid to take on more responsibility, because he was afraid to make mistakes. He is a talented man who could achieve anything in life if he wanted to, but he chooses to stay in his comfort zone and not move to the next level in his life. He is missing a tremendous opportunity to provide a better life for his family and himself, because he is afraid to make changes. He is not growing, and he is stuck on a job for the rest of his life. I hate to think what is going to come to his mind at the end of his career when he looks back and realizes all the opportunities he missed.

Have you ever seen someone who has been on the same job for years? They are comfortable, they do not want more responsibility and they are happy with the wage? These are the people just waiting for their yearly raise to come. They all have one thing in common. They say they are happy with the job and do not need any more responsibility, but they are scared to death to try anything new. Any little change makes them uncomfortable, and they can't handle it. They want to be comfortable. They do not want to be challenged. Where do you think those who never face their fears, never try new things, end up? You probably agree with me that they become stuck in the same situation until they die. When we're doing the same job for more than four years, we become complacent, or we begin to hate it.

133

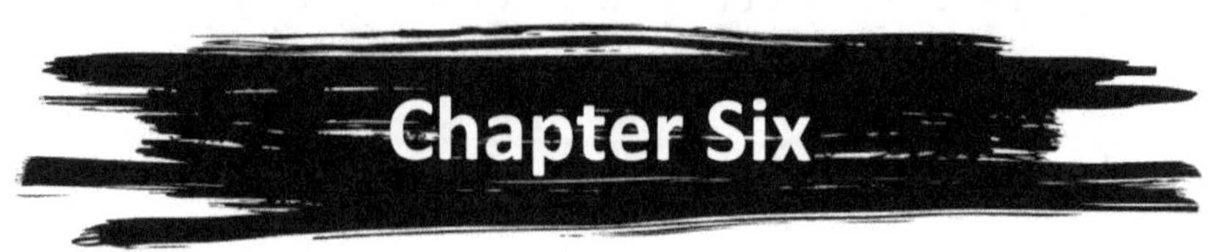

Chapter Six

Expect the Unexpected

In May 2007, I couldn't have felt more blessed. Life had smiled on me in business and family. I felt such a close relationship with God as I had gone from a life of deprivation to the life I had always dreamed of. I felt invincible!

One Saturday evening, to celebrate the birth of my fourth child, "Sheana," we invited some close friends and relatives of my wife, who arrived from New York. I was tending to the barbecue, and my wife tended to all our guests. My wife and I felt very blessed and fortunate that we had built a family together and that we could serve as an example of the American dream. Showing that it is possible to achieve your dreams and no matter what difficulties you face on the road to success, it is important to keep fighting without giving up.

While I was talking with a close friend and grilling, my wife walked over to me while speaking on the phone. I could see from the look of surprise on Fatima's face that this was not an ordinary phone call. She quickly passed me the phone. To my surprise, it was my Aunt Rosa who lived in Spain. It had been a long time since we had spoken, at least six or seven years. My Aunt Rosa is my mother's younger sister. Remember, my mother had raised five siblings along with me, so my aunt and I grew up together. We were like brother and sister, not aunt and nephew. We had a close and loving bond growing up, but distance, combined with years of no communication, separated us. Since it had been so long since we had last spoken, her call was a big surprise.

I thought she was calling because of the birth of my daughter, so I was expecting her to be warm and welcoming. Instead, the phone call was very suspicious and strange. I tried to engage my Aunt in some conversation about the birth of my daughter, Sheana, but I could tell she wasn't listening. Immediately, I could hear in her tone of voice that sounded very peculiar and different, almost as if she was hiding something. It was odd she didn't congratulate us or even acknowledge our new baby girl. I didn't realize it at the time, but she was about to reveal such a dark secret about my mother that would transform my life completely. As she was talking, my gut was telling me something she wasn't saying. There had to be a reason for her call. My first inclination was maybe she wanted money, but I realized her call probably had something to do with my mother, as she was really the only connection we had left. My intuition took over, and without thinking about it, I asked my Aunt Rosa, "Can you believe what my mother is doing?" Immediately, she started crying. The kind of cry that is so powerful that you can't even breathe. As I waited for her to calm down, I had a million ideas racing through my mind. Was my mother seriously ill or injured? Had she been in an accident? Did she kill someone and was she in Jail? Was she alive?

As I looked around, my friends were talking and laughing and enjoying the moment. I realized I needed to take this call in private, so I asked Fatima to take care of the BBQ, so I could figure out what was happening with my mother. Finally, she regained the strength in her voice, and I asked her, "Tell me, what's going on with mother?" She said: "Your mother is dating a guy ten years younger than you."

These were the last words I could ever imagine hearing. As I was growing up, my mother never dated men. She felt she wanted to be there 100 percent for me; therefore, she had no time or energy for other men. Our relationship was so close she never went to the movies or dinner by herself, let alone with a male companion. She sacrificed her personal life for the sake of mine. All I had ever known was my mother's dedication, so I was in shock by my Aunt's revelation. I paused the conversation for a minute or two, trying to assimilate the information I was just given.

At first, I was skeptical of my aunt's accusation. My mother had never communicated any details of this relationship with me. I spoke to her almost every day on the phone, so I would know if she was in a so-called relationship. Not to mention, I had just been to the Dominican Republic two weeks prior. There was no evidence she was dating anyone. She seemed fine everything was the same as always.

"This is impossible, Aunt Rosa. I don't believe it. Why would you say such a thing?"

"Manny, if you don't believe me, then call your uncles. We've been talking, and everyone in the family is worried. We're worried because he is so much younger than her, and what worries us, on top of that he is a married man." A married man? I asked. What she was saying was crazy. I didn't believe it. We are talking about my mother, the woman who sacrificed her life to raise me; the woman who always taught me to do the right thing and who had fought so hard to make her son the man I am today.

"My mother is dating a guy ten years younger than me, and he's married?"

"Yes, and there's one more thing. Everybody in town knows he's taking advantage of her. For months, she's been giving him all kinds of gifts and money, which he's taking and using for his family."

My aunt explained that she and my uncles have tried to talk sense into her to cut off the relationship, but she is not listening. She doesn't care what anyone has to say. Everyone in the family believed she should end that relationship now as it would only bring her pain and suffering.

"Manny, you are the only person who can convince your mother to wake up and realize this is a dangerous relationship. That this guy is taking advantage of her, and you are the only one who can fix it."

At first, I refused to intervene in the relationship because I thought this was a conflict between her and her siblings, and I wanted to stay out of the situation. My aunt pushed on, trying to convince me to get involved: "If you love your mother as much as she loves you, go there, talk to her and make her leave that relationship."

Aunt Rosa told me my mother had turned into a different person since she began dating this guy. She drank and partied. She was wearing clothes that were too young for her age. She was pulling away from the family, rarely talking or socializing. When she got together with her family, she was aggressive and distant. This was not the mother I knew, and this new behavior disturbed me.

Remember, everyone in town knows about my mother. She was so well respected and loved for what she did. She supported people; they came to her for advice and direction. She came from such humble beginnings and overcame such obstacles - everyone looked to her with such respect and admiration. She was considered "The Godmother" to so many people in the town, and no one dared to confront her about her new boyfriend and her new lifestyle.

Aunt Rosa made her final plea: "Manny, she won't listen to any of us. Itis up to you to make her realize this is a dangerous relationship. We've all tried, and no one can convince her otherwise. Your mother loves you so much that you are the only person who can make her realize that this is a mistake. She'll never choose someone else over you."

If this is true, then I knew what I had to do. I promised my aunt that the next day I would fly to the Dominican Republic and figure this out. I assured her I had a surefire way she could never say no to. After hanging up the phone call, I had to take a few minutes alone to digest what I heard. Could my mother, who many considered being just like Mother Teresa, be involved with a guy who is married, with kids and with a man who I saw grow up before my very eyes?

I returned to the party, but my mind was elsewhere than on celebrating Sheana's arrival. I was confused, and I had serious doubts about this revelation. After the guests left for the evening, I sat down and told Fatima about the phone call. She agreed that the right thing to do was to go and investigate the situation for myself. While she packed my suitcase for me, I booked my flight home to the Dominican Republic.

That night, I could only sleep for an hour or two. Everything my aunt told me kept spinning around my mind. I couldn't believe this was happening, especially with my mom. I felt anxious. This was something I had to see with my own eyes. I was confident if any of this was true, I could solve it, and everything would return to normal.

The next day, I made my way to Newark Airport and boarded my flight to the Dominican Republic. As I sat on the plane and looked out the window, my mind drifted. I thought back to my childhood and the sacrifices my mother made for me... was I somehow the cause of her newfound love affair?

I had just been in the DR two weeks ago, and I hadn't noticed anything different. Was I not looking or because I was too focused on growing my business? I thought about the conversation Fatima and my mother had the month prior. My mother commented that she knows of a young guy she'd like to help, providing him with the same support and guidance I received from my mentors. Was this the same man my aunt was talking about?

I thought about how my mother asked me to leave my clothes, my shoes and even my cologne behind during my trips home. She wanted to give to people in need. Was her boyfriend now wearing the new suit jacket I left behind two weeks ago? I grew more suspicious, but my doubts faded. How do you have a conversation with a woman who has given you everything in life, who is now dating a married man almost 30 years younger than her?

Before I knew it, the plane landed, and I was in my rental car on the way home to see my mom. This is a trip I always enjoy, taking in the view of the mountains, rivers and the lushness of the island. But this time, I couldn't pay attention to the beauty of my homeland. I was distracted and thinking about the best way to handle the situation. I wanted to apply the concepts I had learned from my mentor, confident she would make the right decision in a wise and sensible way.

When I finally arrived at the house, I walked through the front door and walked straight into the kitchen. As I predicted, she was surprised to see me. This was the first time I had ever popped in for a unannounced visit. As I went to hug her, I could feel her tension. I could see in her eyes and on her face, she was different. Her hands were shaking, and I got the feeling she knew I was there to talk about her new love affair.

How do you question your most beloved mother? There, she and I were looking at each other face-to-face and uncomfortable with the situation. I had an idea. I asked my mother to make us some coffee. While standing there having our coffee, I tried to relax the situation and made some small talk. After a few minutes of conversation about nothing, I asked my mother to sit down at the table. I had something I needed to ask her.

"Aunt Rosa called yesterday to tell me about something and I want to know if it's true. Are you having an affair with Ramon?"

She responded without hesitation and any sentiment. "Yes."

"Do you know that this guy is married with kids?" "Yes."

"Do you know he is taking advantage of you?"

She defended him. "No, it is nothing like that. He is a really good guy. You just don't know him like I do."

In that moment I realized, everything that my Aunt told me was true. She was a different person. How could that be? How did I not notice this? What happened? "Your family is worried and concerned about you. You need to leave this guy."

She replied one more time without hesitation. "Why should I?" She sat across the table from me, her arms crossed over her chest, defiant about her relationship. She wasn't budging. I reached into my briefcase and found two envelopes. I grabbed a pen and wrote MANNY down on one and RAMON on the other. I was confident in the love she had always shown me and in her promise, I would always be the most important thing in her life. I explained the anguish I felt and the risk she was taking with that relationship. She did not answer and refused to continue the conversation. That's when I placed the envelopes on the table in front of her. "I want you to choose between him or me. Pick one." She stared at me without saying a word while I waited for her to choose the envelope with my name.

Looking back at this moment if I had the opportunity to do this all over again, I would have done things differently. Who am I to put the most important person in my life between the sword and the wall; the woman who gave me life and sacrificed everything for me. At the time, I felt the only option was to have her make the choice of a lifetime, me or him. As she reached for the envelope, I watched her hands, fully expecting her to choose the one labeled MANNY. Instead, she chose RAMON.

At that moment, that millisecond, something so indescribable and life-altering happened, that it took me and my family ten years to recover from it. Never in my life could I have imagined my Mother choosing someone over me. It is difficult for me to express the feeling of abandonment overcoming me at that moment. All my life, I had felt abandoned by my father and now had to relive it for a second time. I wasn't prepared to face it again, especially from the person who I thought loved me above everyone else. Even as I write this, the intensity of these emotions squeezes my heart. It's a feeling I'll never escape, a feeling burned so deep in my mind, I can still feel the fear of that moment. After she made her choice, she stood up, and without eye contact or acknowledgment of her decision, she walked out of the house through the back door. I sat at the kitchen table in shock. I cried. Devastation filled my body, and I experienced the reality of the situation. It was unimaginable and I questioned everything.

Have you ever experienced a situation that made you question everything in life? Why do I exist? What is my purpose in life? Why do so many bad things happen to me? Why am I alive? Why do the people you love most sometimes hurt you?

I had gone through many difficult times in life - many failures. Even before I was born, my father abandoned me I was almost shot and killed by my first wife, the biological mother of my son. I was a failure with God for not completing the seminary. I couldn't complete my studies at the university. I went through innumerable difficulties during my first five years in the United States: I was homeless, eating from garbage cans. Many times, I was discriminated against and rejected because I was an immigrant. All of these were nothing compared to what I was feeling at that moment. After all the hardships I had endured until now made sense because my quality of life improved and it had all been worth it. If life is so vulnerable why do we have faith and believe in ourselves every day? I was not sure I wanted to exist anymore. How do you deal with the rejection of someone you love more than you love yourself?

Life is an incredible journey. You can work so hard and achieve so much that you feel you have it all together and that you can handle anything. Then comes something that hits you so hard that it weakens you to your core.

My Mother's decision also had a physical impact on me. After she left the house, I fell to the ground, unable to stand up, paralyzed. I was in shock, my whole body shook from the sorrow. I could not stop crying. While I was lying there on my mother's kitchen floor, I thought about my wife and children waiting for me at home in the United States. I loved them, they needed me, and they were my reason for being. I had to find the strength and courage to face this challenge that God had placed in my path.

God has shown me that behind great difficulties, there are teachings. Our challenge is to discover what lies behind the failure. That thought gave me the strength to get up.

Stunned, I got up and somehow returned to the airport and boarded the flight back home. I was crying all the way, thinking about what had happened and trying to find a justification. I wanted to talk to no one. I remember that people looked at me as if I was crazy. I must have had a vacant look on my face when I went through the immigration security checkpoint. They almost stopped me because I could barely answer the immigration officer's questions.

Somehow, I made the drive back home. I vaguely remember that my wife helped me to lie down in bed... I don't think I said a single word to my wife when I got home that night. I felt a pain in my back, and I could hardly move my legs. This catastrophic event affected me so deeply that it physically impaired my basic motor functions.

The next morning, I couldn't get out of bed. I felt a crushing pain in my body, like I was carrying the entire world on my shoulders. It felt horrible, the worst I've ever felt. I could not move my legs or my arms, nor could I get out of bed. Fatima was so scared; she had never seen me lifeless like that before. I was in such pain, and she was worried for my life, so she called the ambulance to take me to the emergency room.

At the hospital, the doctors couldn't understand where my pain originated. They gave me CAT Scans and X-Rays; they tested everything and couldn't find anything that was causing my pain. Even the strongest of pain tranquilizers couldn't relieve the pain in my body. I stayed in the hospital for a few days under observation, but my situation did not improve. The doctors sent me home because there was nothing further, they could do for me. I laid on my back, unable to move and my body full of pain. My children had always looked at me as a hero, now I was practically paralyzed. I could see from the concern on Fatima's face I was suffering, and so was she.

I shared with Fatima and my family the horrible choice my mother made. While they comforted me with my physical pain, the real pain was in my heart and soul. Reflecting on that moment, little did I understand that the love for my mom became the next obstacle in my life. It all felt temporary, that soon I would wake up as if nothing had happened, I had hoped that everything would continue as before.

The days, weeks and months passed, and while the pain in my back and body receded, the pain in my heart multiplied. Many things changed. I felt great fatigue, losing my energy and my passion for life. I felt I was carrying a heavyweight of guilt and sadness, so much that it manifested in severe pain in my upper back, neck, and shoulders. I felt useless, my thoughts became blurred, and I moved drifted due to the almost unbearable pain.

I didn't want to leave the house anymore. I isolated myself from everyone. I'd sit in the backyard by myself for hours and hours every day, so I didn't have to interact with my family and friends. I went so far as changing my cell phone number so no one, not even my customers, could contact me.

I sold all my rental properties for prices well below their value. One of the rental properties I purchased for $200,000 a year prior, I sold at a significant loss for only $35,000. I stopped caring about being rich and so-called successful. In my mind, I felt I should give up all my assets, abandon everything I worked so hard for to achieve. No one could understand what was happening, especially not Fatima. She would challenge my rash decisions and question my reckless behavior, but I didn't listen to a word she had to say. I sold all my properties, destroyed my businesses and my reputation and everything we had worked so hard for to achieve. I wanted to disappear into a black hole. I felt as if I was dead inside. My mother gave me life and now she delivered what felt like a fatal blow, a death sentence.

Little by little, I lost all the passion for living. The desire to work hard and maintain my level of success completely disappeared. Having money did not matter anymore. In a frenzy of activity, I gave away everything I had accumulated. I donated all the assets of my businesses to my church. I gave away all the tools, vans and work trucks to my employees, valued at hundreds of thousands of dollars. One after another, I closed all my businesses and destroyed the legacy I had worked so hard to create.

Steve, my mentor, was worried. Before this transformation in my life, we would talk practically every day. I could only keep him away so long. He would stop by my house, asking to see me, worried that something serious had happened. Fatima would tell him I was not home, but he knew I was avoiding him. Steve was one of the most important people in my life, and I didn't want to see or talk to him ever again. Avoiding all contact with friends and family, I disappeared completely from my old life. Psychologically, I wanted to be poor again, and through my actions, I succeeded. In a few years, there I was, poorer than ever.

This was not a conscious thought or decision I made. Honestly, I did not realize what I was doing. I was lost in my inner pain. I wanted to withdraw from the world while I was in a state of poverty, and what is worse, I took my wife and children with me. I was without my business, without my property and any passion for life. What do you do when you lose everything? When the will to live is gone, when your life no longer makes sense? I felt myself die inside. Unconsciously, I wanted to die.

Throughout my life, despite all the adversities put in front of me, I had always looked for a way to solve my problems. I had always faced my challenges without fear, without doubt for even a moment I would achieve everything I set out to do. I had shrunk down to the shadow of that strong man, the person who rose every morning to challenge nature; the guy who pushed past his comfort zone; the one who challenged the world and never saw the impossible. There I was, dead inside and the flame in my heart, a dying ember. I sat back and watched what was happening around me but could do nothing to stop my erratic behavior. Why was I destroying my life? I loved my wife and children; my family was the truest and realest thing I ever had. Why was I putting their lives at risk? I knew at some level, what I was doing to my family was wrong, but I could not escape the mental pain I was under. I continued this dark road for almost five years. I was driving without headlights, without guidance.

As my life continued to spiral downward, another even more disastrous idea occurred. One day I decided to move my family to Trenton, New Jersey. Trenton at that time was a city with the highest crime rates in the United States. Now you may be wondering why I want to move from a house near to the beach in a safe neighborhood to a city with high crime. At that moment I did not know why, but later I understood that I wanted to lose my life, I wanted for someone to kill me.

My wife resisted, although she never used to say anything about what I decided, but I knew it was a bad idea. She knew I was struggling dealing with the tragedy, but she was determined to fight with me for this decision. She tried to convince me not to make the move, but it didn't change my mind. I packed my bags, and I was ready to go. I would go alone if I had to, but I would move to Trenton with or without them. I don't know why I acted like this. I knew I was hurting my family and, most importantly I was placing my entire family in danger but at that moment, I didn't mind.

We left our house near the beach, packed some of our belongings and made the move. Leaving all our furniture and belongings abandoned, I wanted nothing to remind me of my past. It seemed like I was running away from something, and, I think I was running away from myself and everything that reminded me of my past life. I remember my wife was crying, and my children were uncomfortable. The house was in a terrible neighborhood, and many days we had to fall to the floor because we heard gunshots outside. There were moments when people would get killed right in front of our house. We had to keep the curtains closed at all times. The windows of my car were broken several times, and the tires crushed. We didn't have much money to buy groceries. We had very little furniture because we left everything in the old house. We ended up in a worse situation than when we came to the United States. I had destroyed our lives. You can imagine how I felt when seeing my family going through so many difficulties and I could do nothing. That feeling of helplessness I can only explain to you by mentioning a similar situation, but it's like seeing someone you love so much falling off a cliff and you are standing still without moving to help them. That's how I felt. I watched what I had caused, but it was like I could do nothing, I felt as if I was a ghost and I could only see what was happening, but I could not intervene.

Sometimes at night, I would go for a walk and not pay attention to traffic when I crossed the street. I walked at night when the streets were dangerous. I was wandering through life like a sleepwalker. I lived in a haze of misery. I was so lost I barely have memories of those dark years. Most of what I remember today comes from the memories of my wife and children. I was lost to myself and the world. I was a shell of a man, walking, talking, and breathing, but dead inside.

Today, as I write this book and think about that moment, I look for the reason that would explain my actions. What I have noticed is that I moved to Trenton because I wanted to die. I could not take my life. I was looking for someone to take it for me. My wife cried silent tears every day. She used to go to church to get free food and clothes for the children. Before, I had planned to retire at forty. Now here I was in our worst situation yet. We had no hope, no possibilities, and no passion or desire for life. There was a dark cloud inside me and about my life, and my family lived in dangerous conditions because of me. Here I was lost, without purpose, with no intention to take any risk, to find a job, to be someone again. I was sitting in a chair wondering what had happened to me, not understanding why and how I will get out of this darkness.

Have you ever been in a situation and you wanted to leave? You probably even knew what you should do, but did not take any action to move forward? That was me. I knew I had to do something. I knew I could go back to my mentor and start my business again. I knew I could ask for help from the people who loved me. However, I sat in my house every day to watch the day go by. Instead, every action I made moved us further in the wrong direction.

Most people know what they need to change in their life, what behaviors need to be changed and what skills are needed to achieve their goals, but because we want to be comfortable, we are not willing to make the changes and take any risks. We rather want to stay in the comfort zone because it is the easy thing to do.

One afternoon, my wife was watching television with my youngest daughter, Sheana, sitting on the floor. While I was sitting in the backyard, like every other day, watching life go by. She called me: "Manny, Manny, please come here. I want you to see something. Come quickly." I saw a psychologist on a television program that talked about the symptoms of depression. He was describing the behaviors and symptoms I had been showing. In that moment, everything made sense. I finally understood what was wrong with me. For the past five years, I had sunk into a deep depression unnoticed. With that realization, a little light began to shine in my life.

Now I had a name and a face for the enemy, depression. I could begin to find a solution to this problem. I thought about how the depression forced me make decisions I was not proud of. At that moment, Fatima and I decided to get help. I was determined to transform my life one more time. To start all over again. As I was reflecting that moment, the love of my mother destroyed my life, but this time, the love of my kids, my wife and the desire to transform my life again gave me the motivation to find a solution to my depression. We found a psychologist near our house in Trenton, NJ. He was an expert in hard depression, and I was sure he would give the diagnostic I needed. I made an appointment. He made me come every day for a couple of weeks. I had to explain and share with him all the events of my life, from my childhood growing up, all the situations, good and bad that I had been through. I also shared with him what I thought caused my depression. As we finished the sessions, he gave me insights that opened my eyes completely. He helped me to understand that depression came not only from the rejection of my mother. The depression was the accumulation of events I have been through in my entire life. The meeting with my mother had awoken a deep depression that laid dormant within me. A silent killer.

The diagnosis from the doctor:

"Manny, you have a hard depression,"

"What is hard depression?" I asked.

"You are not able to identify your own unique needs and taking steps to meet them — for example make time to do things you normally do, and perform activities to keep your life going. Your emotions and physical reactivity have been siphoned off, draining you of the ability to look after yourself."

While he was explaining the reasons behind my behaviors and actions, I felt some type of relief and understanding for them.

"Doctor, what are my options?" I asked.

"Manny, you only have two options. One is quicker than the other. With one you will be feeling relief faster than the other. I will explain both to you and I want you to think about it before you make a final decision."

The first option is to take antidepressants, and in a few weeks, you will start feeling better. You will experience happiness and joy in your life again. But you need to know you will need to take this medication every day for the rest of your life.

The second option is to find something you used to love doing in the past and do it again. This option will be difficult to achieve and it will take you a long time to recover from your depression. I do not guaranty this option will be the right thing to do. He also mentioned his patients mostly take antidepressants because they will fix the problem faster. I went home with an important decision to make. I had to choose if I wanted to take the faster or the longer way to transform my life.

I chose to not take any medication; instead, I looked for motivation within. For the next couple days, Fatima and I sat down laying out all the different jobs and activities I've done in my life. I was determined to find my passion again. As you know by now, I was not willing to take the fast road if there's a hard way. I needed to challenge myself and find a complete escape. I knew a temporary solution would only delay the depression; I needed to end it.

We sat at the table across from each other. We placed a piece of paper on top of the table, Fatima grabbed a pen, and she was ready to write all the activities I had done or worked on for the past 20 years of my life. She asked me, "Manny, think about all the different jobs you have done here in America."

"I worked in landscaping, factories, the car wash, constructions, rental properties…."

While I listed them, I didn't feel any interest in doing any of these jobs. After spending a couple hours brainstorming, we came to a dead-end. We looked at each other thinking about what we would do now. In my mind, I thought it would be easy. We sat there for hours thinking about all the different possibilities with no luck. Then, Fatima had a brilliant idea. I think she noticed I was avoiding doing anything that reminds me of my past life here in America. She asked me: "Why don't we look for things you would do when you were in the Dominican Republic?"

Ah! "It is a great idea." I used to love working at Burger King, I said.

At that moment, when I mentioned Burger King, my heart felt a different sensation, and at that moment, I knew this was the right thing for me to do. Honestly, I had never considered a comeback to work at Burger King, but it sounded interesting, and it caught my attention. I loved working at Burger King. I was passionate about my work when I worked there. I thought it would be a good place to start, but I didn't know how to begin.

I immediately picked the phone to call the doctor. I wanted to share the news. I knew medication worked for many people, but I wanted to apply the power of discomfort in my life. I wanted to be strong again, plus I knew I could count on the support of my wife and children. I don't recommend for anyone, not to follow the doctor recommendations, but in my case, it was a personal commitment, and I owed it to my family. I have struggled my entire life; I've faced many obstacles, why shouldn't I face one more? It is never too late to start over again, to try a new venture, to start a new job, to direct or redirect your life.

I felt this time I was going in the right direction. I was not doing anything to prove to my father what he missed, or to prove to anyone they were wrong. I felt different I knew of my thoughts and behaviors, and most importantly, I was doing it for my family.

The relief finally came. I was ready to leave that hopeless place. I asked my wife and children to sit at the table, and while we were sitting, I looked at everyone one by one, with tears in my eyes. I asked them to please forgive me. I had disappointed them, and I promised them I would fight to get back to that man I was before, and I also promised them that I would get us away from this dangerous neighborhood to a safer place. For the next couple days, I spent hours thinking about how I was going to join Burger King.

I was determined to rebuild my life. I knew the route I chose would be difficult and uncomfortable, but I knew I had to challenge myself every day to become the person I deserved. If not, I could not rekindle my passion for life.

 If you've been successful once, you can be successful twice. I thought. I needed to build a new circle of friends and, most importantly, I would not be afraid to ask for help. I felt alive again, and I felt hopeful. I was positive throughout the process. There was a way to get my life back, and I was willing to do whatever it took to get there. I wanted my family to feel proud of me again, but I was not afraid to start over. If you are afraid to start over, or challenge yourself, to get out of your comfort zone, most likely you won't be able to transform your life.

For the next couple of days, my wife and I tried to discover a game plan for me to find a job at Burger King. This time, my excitement was different. In the past, I wanted to be successful because I wanted to be rich and retire young. Now I wanted to be successful because I wanted to help others who suffered in life. I wanted them to see possibilities in my story. I knew I would have to start from the bottom again, but I was not afraid to climb. The journey seemed long and impossible a few months ago. Now it just seemed long. Soon it will be a reality. Successful people can lose their fortune and rebuild their lives over again. We have heard these stories thousands of times. I knew I could do it. I would be another comeback story and with wife was by my side all the time working to help me overcome my depression this was undoubtedly possible.

One morning I was about to give up and go to a local restaurant to apply for a team member position. I couldn't find a job. Then I remembered Armando, who worked for Burger King. He would inspect my restaurants, but he also oversaw franchise relations back in the Dominican Republic. He knew me, and we spent a lot of time together working in the restaurants. I immediately grabbed my computer and searched his name on Google. I was pleasantly surprised to see he was still working for the company. Not only did he work there, but he was also the president of the Latin America stores.

My heart was beating faster. I was excited, and at the same time, I was wondering if he would remember me. It had been over twelve years since I had last seen him, but I didn't let that stop me. Doubts filled my mind. My wife asked: "He is now an important man; why would he take the time to help you or even answer an email?", but I was confident that he would help me like my other mentors in life. After a few minutes, I went to type an email, which would be the beginning of my new life. I wrote a message and sent it to him. To my surprise, he responded within five minutes. He didn't return my email; he called me. He remembered me, and we talked for about an hour to catch up with our lives in recent years. Then, I went into the reason I was contacted him. I asked if he would help me get a job with Burger King here in America. He said: "Of course, let me see what I can do, and I'll have someone contact you tomorrow."

Here again, I was about to transform my life because I had the courage to ask for help. If you ask others for help, most people are willing to help you. We just need to have the courage to ask. Most of the time, we are stuck in life for not asking someone to help us. There were many days I wanted to pick up the phone and ask my mentor, Steve for help. I did not, because I was willing to start all over again. If I want to transform my life, I must do something I have not done. I disconnected from our call feeling very excited. This was my opportunity to start over again, to recover and transform my life. I was ready to return to the game and fight for my present and the future of my family. People don't realize that people in power and leadership roles - at least those who weren't born into them - got there by asking for help. They remember the exact time they changed their life - that's why they are eager to help. If you want to be a journalist, find your favorite writer and shoot him an email, ask him for help. If you want to be a chef, find your favorite restaurant and ask to speak with the head chef. You learn by doing, but you also learn by asking.

Every so often, life hits you hard. It can take you down a dark path where you fall and lose everything, yourself included, a path that seems endless. These difficult times hurt. They erase the good within you, the memories of prosperity and happiness. Everything seems bad. None of this matters if you have the desire to live a better life and the will to start over again, to make sacrifices and be uncomfortable, do the things you do not want to do. Stop crying and take action. The great thing about being at the bottom is you have nothing to lose and everything to gain. You can't go any further down, but like being on the bottom of the ocean, you can feel the sand, and you can push yourself up. The only way now is up. Think of your body floating through the water, you gain momentum. You propel faster. The smallest action you take can give a positive result. Like a push, or a ripple that can transform into a wave that carries you further with each moment in time.

I found myself at the bottom, what else could I lose? I realized anything that changes in my life would be beneficial for me. It is never too late to start over. You can always change the behaviors you know preventing you from reaching your goals. For me, it was my depression, losing desire, the unwillingness to move forward. In that moment I thought about everything Steve taught me.

If I were to change my life, I needed to become the person I was before my depression. To help me get there, I needed to find that person who would help me and show me what I could not see to achieve success again. It was time for me to search for a new mentor.

I worked for Burger King again. Throughout this process, I met Matt, he helped me to work through my depression without even knowing he was doing it. He challenged me, helped me raise my expectations, to trust others, work smarter, and most importantly, to believe in myself again. Finally, I was excited again about the future, my future and I easily identified that I wanted to obtain a role within the American cooperation. I was working as a restaurant general manager, but I kept the vision firmly implanted in my mind. I think when Matt told me I was not ready to lead multiple restaurants; it opened a desire in me to prove him wrong. I am not sure about you, but if someone told me I couldn't do something, the desire to compete and show them anything is possible takes over. Some people believe the naysayers.

At this point I knew I had some challenges to face. I still had a very heavy accent. I am Latino. I have grammar issues and the last time I worked in Burger King was in my country 12 years ago. This did not sit well with everyone, especially my immediate supervisor. He did everything possible to get me fired. He didn't train me or give any feedback. He falsified numbers to make me look bad. He didn't want me to be successful. Even with all these challenges I had to face, I did not give up; I pushed myself to the limit. I believe he felt threatened, but all his opposition only drove me to work harder and further challenge myself. Instead of hurting me, he unintentionally helped. I used his negativity to fuel my success. I quickly realized that in the corporate world, I had to work much harder than the average American to compete, much less get ahead. I worked fourteen-hour days. I studied company operations manuals, so I could become an expert in operations. I dedicated time to read books on leadership and people management so I could understand people's behaviors. I would read a book every two weeks to improve my knowledge. I applied the knowledge my mentor has taught me, I was obsessed over learning. I wanted to be ready when the opportunity presented itself. It was a new environment for me. In the past, I owned my own businesses and others would follow my directions. Now, I had to convince the people to do what I wanted them to do and follow my vision. It was not an easy thing to master.

I would often work double shifts. I had to be careful driving home because I sometimes fell asleep behind the wheel. I was working hard, many times without a day off. I was tired, but it didn't matter because I was working towards my goal. My goal was to climb the corporate ladder and land at the top. I wanted to make my wife and children proud of me again. I didn't want them to see me as a hopeless and depressed father.

After a few months of working as a manager, I approached the director of the operations from Burger King. I had chosen Matt to be my mentor; he just didn't know it yet. I saw him as my role model. He was a very wise man, a fantastic leader, and I wanted to learn from him. If you want to be the best, you must learn from the best. He was visiting my restaurant, and he was very happy with the significant improvements I had made to the operations in the short time I had been there. He asked me: "What can I do for you?" Here was my opportunity to connect with him and build a relationship of coaching and teaching I envisioned from him.

I responded, "There is something I would love you to do for me. From the first day I met you, I admired you, and my goal is to be like you one day. I want to eventually take your position, but I know I need to be prepared. I want to know if you could spend an hour a week with me so I can learn from you. I can come to wherever you are, and I promise to do it on my day off." He smiled and responded, "I can't spend an hour each week with you because I have a lot going on, but what I can do is spend one day each month with you. We can tour restaurants, and I'm sure you can learn a lot about what I do." He thought I could never reach this level, with all the weaknesses and challenges I had. I would not let how he felt stop me. This was a huge step for me to take, but I was not afraid to face any obstacles or challenges that stood in my way. I believe you can do anything their heart desires if they are strong enough to withstand the resistance of human nature. Matt's answer was exactly what I wanted to hear. I grew excited and saw my plan getting one step closer to my goal. I had the opportunity to learn from someone who has already achieved what I want I felt very fortunate to have received help from others, and to have had the opportunity to help others.

I didn't feel alone, and that was gratifying. I wasn't afraid to ask for help, and someone was willing to help me. His answer was the best news I had received in a long time. I couldn't wait to get home to share the news with my family.

 When you can meet someone who already has what you want, you need to take advantage of the moment. Seek advice, ask questions and most importantly, set up a meeting with this person. Remember they know how to get to the place you want to be. Sometimes we have the opportunity to meet someone who can change your life or even guide you in the right directions and we don't take advantage of this opportunity. You must look for these people who are there, sometimes they are near you, and you never have taken the time to notice. I personally looked around for people who have a higher level of thoughts. I want to learn as much as I can. When I was kid, I always wanted to be smarter, but now that I have grown, I ask for wisdom. I want to be wise. To be wise, you need to be humble, face your fears and ask for advice from those individuals that achieved what you want to achieve.

 Over the next year, we spent a day each month together. Sometimes I had to drive four hours to see him on my day off, paying for gas and other expenses on those trips. It didn't bother me though, because I knew the sacrifice would pay off. I learned so much from the meetings. I learned a set of new skills and discovered talent I never knew I had.

One day I thought I was ready to grow, so I asked him what I would need to do to grow in the corporate environment. I felt I was ready to take the next step. He answered: "There is not much that you can accomplish until you improve your English." I thought about that. I said, "My talent, experiences, and drive to succeed don't matter?" His answer was not what I wanted to hear. He said: "In corporate America, if you don't speak English well, and you struggle with grammar, people won't trust you. They will get a bad impression and doubt your intelligence. They won't respect you. When you go for an interview, they'll notice immediately. I recommend you don't waste your time and energy on this, focus on what you can do today."

His answer deflated me. I started to doubt my ability to grow and achieve my goals in a corporate setting. How do you react when someone tells you can't do something? I had been dreaming about this opportunity to grow for months. I made sacrifices and spent my own money for the sole purpose of growing within the company. I was thankful for all the time he had spent with me. What I learned from him helped me to feel I could achieve any opportunity, but now he was telling me it was impossible.

I asked another question. "To be an area supervisor, do I need to speak perfect English?" "No," he answered. "Your interaction with people at the corporate level would be minimal, and if you needed to send an email, I could correct the grammar." You must seize an opportunity when it is presented. And, at this moment, I didn't have what I wanted, but I knew this was one step closer to my dream. Life doesn't give us what we want immediately, but it gives us what we need. For me, at this point, I needed to become an area supervisor.

Matt was not only very smart but also kind. He knew I had the talent to do whatever I wanted in life, no matter the opportunity. He was just as happy getting to know me as I was getting to know him. I believed what he told me about how difficult it would be for me to grow in the corporate arena, but I knew it would be a challenge I would face one day. I wasn't afraid, and I knew I was getting ahead of myself. This was not the right moment to ask him this question; I was way ahead of my possibilities, but at the same time, he made me see my limitations. If I work on overcoming this obstacle, when the opportunity arrives, I will be ready. When we have challenges, we need to face, or skills we need to learn, procrastination can hurt us. I knew I would never stop having an accent in English, but I knew it could get better. In that moment, something Steve had taught me came to mind. I needed to prepare for the opportunity to come, because one day when the opportunity came knocking at my door, I needed to be ready to say hello.

I decided to face the challenges in front of me now and deal with the future when the time came. But at the same time, I prepared for it. I needed to continue building a strong foundation, to prove I would be a great candidate for a higher position in the corporate hierarchy. His words of caution only fueled me to work harder and prove him wrong. When you have a challenge in front of you, there are two ways to see it—put yourself down and give up or find the solution and move forward. It's that simple.

There is one thing I have learned about myself over the years, when you tell me I can't do something, I push myself and make sure I get it done. There is not much I accept as impossible or improbable. I had overcome bigger challenges in my life. This was just one more obstacle for me to overcome. By the end of our discussion, I was no longer deflated. I was filled with the fire to succeed.

Within a few months, they promoted me to area supervisor. Along with the position, I received a considerable raise. Finally, I could move my family out of Trenton to a nicer home in a safer neighborhood. During that week, I took my family out to a nice restaurant to celebrate. It had been a while since we could eat at an expensive restaurant. It was a happy occasion and a turning point for us. My children saw their father as a hard-working, successful man that was no longer sad and depressed. It felt great to treat them to a nice evening - to smile, be happy, show them my love and affection; to let them know how important they are. These happy moments shared with loved ones make life worth living. I realized a year ago I was living in darkness, but with the love and help of my family, I was now in a good place, feeling alive again, and able to express and share my love and appreciation for them. I had received my list of assigned restaurants and signed my offer letter, but just a couple days later, I received some heartbreaking news. They were in the process of selling the company, and because of this, they could not follow through with my promotion.

At this moment, I couldn't believe what I was hearing. I had been working extremely hard for the past year, and when I finally made it to my next opportunity, fate steps in and takes it away. Here I was again, head to head with a difficult challenge. How could I tell my family we would not be moving out of our horrible situation? That for the promotion I had sacrificed and worked so hard for fell through? I did not understand how I would break this news to them. I learned from Steve to find a solution for your challenges. He always said "If there's a challenge, there's a solution - you need to think from another perspective, another point of view." After working that day, I went for a walk in the park. I was disappointed but like my mother always said, something good will come out of this situation.

Even though this was a setback, I was unwilling to give up. I looked for other opportunities before I let my family know I had not received the promotion. I looked with other franchises and remembered my old boss from the Dominican Republic who was working Burger King in New Mexico. I contacted him for help. After a few phone calls and a trip to New Mexico, I could secure a new position. I was hired as an area manager. I moved my entire family to a new state. It was a giant change for us, but a welcomed one. We moved to a great neighborhood, and my children adapted easily to new schools and made new friends. We were finally away from constant crime and daily fear for our well-being. No more waking up to gunshots and crime scenes. No more worrying about the safety of my children. No more Trenton.

I oversaw six restaurants in New Mexico. I liked my new boss; he was very approachable and supportive. We developed a close relationship and became friends. Over the year I spent in that position, our families grew close, and we spent many weekends together.

While working in New Mexico, my old mentor Matt from Burger King called with an offer for a new opportunity to come work with him at Dunkin Donuts. I was ecstatic at the thought of working with him again. I accepted the position without hesitation. I would manage 14 restaurants in Philadelphia. The offer doubled my current salary, so I left New Mexico much easier. I packed up my family and made the move back east. It was a culture shock for my family. We had grown familiar with New Mexico and enjoyed life there, but this was an opportunity I could not pass up because it allowed me to advance one step closer to my goal of becoming a Director of Operations for a major corporation.

I knew working with him again and being surrounded by his guidance and influence would help to get me there. It was just a matter of time. I created a list of five things I needed to accomplish. First, I needed to learn as much as I could from my mentor. Second, I needed to read books to improve my knowledge so I could become an expert on leadership. Third, I needed to build relationships with the surrounding influencers. Four, I needed to improve my English language skills and five, I needed to be persistent and patient. If I focused on these five principles, I would accomplish my goal of becoming the director of operations for a major corporation.

I remember what Steve taught me. "When preparation and opportunity combine, people normally call it good luck. Prepare yourself, work at reinforcing your strengths, discover new talents and skills and others will not ignore you."

Now I know I needed to work smart, not hard. For the past two years I have been working hard, now is the time for me to work smart, to develop my strengths and grow as much as possible. Having a plan makes life much easier. The first thing I understood was that if I wanted to be successful, I needed to build an outstanding team. So, I dedicated a year studying how to build a great team. I read books, articles, and searched the internet for information. I became obsessed with building a great team. I knew if I mastered team building, it would make the difference in my career. With the right team, you can influence them to see your vision. With good leadership and a team aligned with your vision, achieving success is a foregone conclusion. I didn't want my team to do only what I told them; I wanted to convince them to believe in what I believed. I wanted to develop the ability to discover talent in others and help them see what they could not see for themselves. Managing people is an art. Building a great team is an art. Creating people hungry to succeed and share your vision is an art. I wanted to master these skills. I was applying what Steve taught me, "Master your strengths so that others ignore your weaknesses." When I heard this for the first time, I didn't value it as much as I do now. I felt that Steve was preparing me for today. I spent almost my entire life trying to master my weakness, looking for ways to overcome my weaknesses. Through the teachings of my mentors, and my own experiences, I realized it was a waste of time.

When I started at the Dunkin Donuts, the owner was on the verge of losing his restaurants. Corporate had already closed a few of them because of poor operational performance. I took over 14 locations, and within six months, stabilized operations for all of them. We passed all inspections with an "A" rating, and all the positive results were because I could build an amazing team. Sales, profit, and guest satisfaction increased. The owner was thrilled. I was happy because I proved the power of building a great team. With this experience, I felt ready to use my talents at a larger corporation. I would not allow my imperfect English, heavy accent and grammar to hold me back. I was ready for a change, I was hungry, and I felt this time I would do whatever it took to achieve my goal. I prepared myself for a couple of years and now I felt I was ready to accomplish my goal. At that moment, I was impressed how I overcame my depression and the burning desire of being a successful man came to me again.

In 2012, I made the move to Georgia to work for Church's Chicken Corporation as an area supervisor. During the interview, they gave me the choice of three cities and asked where I would like to move. I asked which was the worst market where were the most challenges? They responded, Columbus, Georgia. I immediately replied this was the market I wanted to run. My interviewers were surprised by my answer. They had never had a candidate decide where they wanted to move based the worst market available. Most people make their choices based on other criteria, not least of which is the area with the minimal problems, but if you know by now, I never run from a challenge or the feeling of discomfort. They were intrigued and wanted to see how I would perform. I was ready to astound them. I had become a master in the power of discomfort and building great teams. I had also become an expert at overcoming adversity. I was driven by a desire to achieve excellence. It was the story of my life.

 I went into an area where everyone predicted I would fall in the trail. This was an African-American market and neighborhood. I was the only Latino in any of the restaurants. Most of the restaurants were in high-crime areas. The employees were unhappy to come to work. Sales were down; the restaurants had many opportunities for training, operations, guest service, and theft to name a few.

With my goal in mind, I implemented my plan. I worked hard, but I also worked smart - the key to success. I intended on accomplishing all I needed to within a year and move up to a higher position. I was not willing to stay there for more than a year. I faced many challenges, and I made changes quickly. I changed out 80 percent of the managers because of poor performance and developed all the restaurant general manager replacements through internal promotions. I provided hope and growth opportunities for the people working for me. We built an amazing team. After six months, our results were incredible. Members of the leadership team visited the market, impressed with the turnaround. Sales, profit, and guest satisfaction were up. Turnover increased, and complaints decreased. I was doing what I did best, building a great team that shared the same vision.

Within a year, my area was one of the top performers after years of sitting at the bottom of the list. My team earned bonuses for the first time. I had proven what I was capable of. People were paying attention, and I was attracting notice from the head office. Over time, I gained a reputation for affecting positive change and solid leadership. I was ready to move to a higher position at the corporate head office. I knew it wouldn't be easy to earn the director's position, but I wanted the chance. I was not afraid and feeling confident. I had been preparing for the role for over three years.

During my first month in the market, there was a cook in one restaurant named Copper. As I was walking into the kitchen, I noticed he was cooking chicken correctly and I immediately reached into my pocket to get a recognition card. I wrote a nice message recognizing Copper for the great work he was doing. After I gave him the card, he stopped working and walked out the back door. I didn't know what was going on; I did not understand why he left after I give him a recognition card. Who does not want to be recognized? With many doubts in my mind and trying to understand what just happened, I went outside to look for Copper. He was by the dumpster crying. I apologized to him if I said or did anything that made him uncomfortable. He responded "Manny, I am 32 years old, this is the first time I have received recognition from someone in my life. I am sorry that I am crying but I cannot contain my emotions." It allowed me to understand the power of recognition, and I used Copper's opportunity to motivate my team.

In a few weeks, a position for Director of Operations was coming available. It required overseeing 90 restaurants in "The Valley" in Texas. The current director had been in place for over 10 years, and he was about to leave. My supervisor told me the company was looking to offer me the position. This would be the fulfillment of the goal I had set for myself. I was extremely excited, and my wife and I looked for houses in the area. We were preparing ourselves to be ready once the position became available. My plan was coming reality.

While all of this was happening, the president of the company resigned. They hired a replacement, someone I had admired in my past life when I worked at Burger King. We had had little contact, but the little I saw of him left a great impression on me. He was someone I felt I would like to have as a mentor one day if we had the chance to work together again. Now here he was, being hired as the new President for Church's Chicken. I was happy to see him come aboard.

The time came when the Director of Operations for the Texas market was terminated. It was time to select his replacement. My supervisor contacted me. He said, "Manny, the new executive vice-president and the vice-president of operations want to meet with you." My heart leaped. I thought, "Oh my God, I can't believe I am about to fulfill my dream!" I had been waiting for this day for a few years to come and I had worked tirelessly to achieve it. I prepared myself for their visit. I made sure all my restaurants were ready and made sure there would be no surprises. I spoke with each of my managers to prepare them for the visit. I told them, "Don't be nervous. I'm not asking you to do anything you haven't done before. Just be yourselves and do the same job you do every day." I wanted them to feel confident and take pride in all they had achieved. I wanted them to know I trusted them and was proud of them. It helped them to feel more comfortable with the visit.

The day came, and the vice-presidents toured my restaurants with me. They were impressed with our results and paid compliments to the restaurant teams. They were happy with the energy and engagement of everyone in the restaurants. While touring, we all drove in the same car. The Executive Vice President was friendly and asked about my family. He gave me his compliments on the market and all we had accomplished. I felt very comfortable in their company. During our conversation, he asked me a question.

He said: "If you had to do this all over again and come back to Columbus and find the same challenges, what would you do differently?"

I replied without thinking, saying, "I wouldn't do anything differently. I would do everything the same because I have been so successful."

At that moment, my supervisor turned around from the front seat and looked at me. Everyone stopped talking, and I felt like a kid that said something bad in front of grown-ups. I was embarrassed. I did not know why, but I was. The answer I gave was the wrong one. We drove for about 10 minutes, but it felt like an hour. All the excitement drained away. From the look on everyone's face, I knew my answer was not what they expected.

Once we arrived at the last restaurant, my boss pulled me aside. He told me, "Manny, forget about this position for now; you are not ready."

"Why?" I asked. He answered my question with a question.

He asked me: "Have you ever made any mistakes while you're here?"

I said, "Oh yeah, I have made many mistakes."

He asked me: "Would you handle your mistakes differently?"

I said, "Of course, I would." At that moment, it all clicked in my head, I understood the mistake I had made. I couldn't believe I failed at something so simple. I also couldn't believe a single response to a question would determine my future.

I asked him another question. "Why is the answer to this question so important?"

He said, "If you wouldn't do anything different, that means you're not learning from your mistakes. You would probably make the same mistakes many times. Once you are at the director's level, you have to learn from your mistakes."

I was disappointed with myself, but I was also not happy that a single answer would prevent me from gaining this opportunity. I went home having learned a big lesson. It was a perfect scenario for me to ask myself the two question my mentor Steve asked me what I did well and what I can do differently. Obviously, you can notice I was not asking these two questions during this time. After that day, I ask myself this every day. I learned so much during this time. One question transformed the way I saw things.

As I thought about it more, another lesson from my mentor came to mind. Be patient. I didn't get that director's position. I continued working in my market for the next couple of months until another opportunity came along. Another position was open in San Antonio, Texas. To understand how my answer pushed me back, I was not even considered for an interview. It felt as if that one question derailed my future. I knew it wouldn't be easy, and I was prepared for that. I knew I had to work harder than any American to be recognized. I knew I had to master my strengths if I wanted to be noticed. For all these reasons, I waited for the right opportunity. Sometimes in live things to not happen when you want them to, they happen when you least expect them.

At the end of 2014, I was ready to interview for the position of director of operations excellence. It was a better position than the prior ones. However, this time, I was not willing to take any risks. I needed to prepare myself. Four candidates were interviewing for the same position. They were conducting two rounds of interviews. The first round, they would interview all four candidates. The best two would advance to the second round. From there, they would decide on the best candidate. I would interview with the same two vice presidents I had given my disastrous answer to before.

I asked a few people to help me prepare for the interview process, including my boss. I spent hours researching the position. I also planned for my first 30, 60, 90 days, six months, and one year. I investigated what makes this position successful and what challenges this position was facing, and I also planned to overcome the obstacles. This time, I would go in prepared. I would not miss this opportunity to have my dream become a reality again . Being overconfident did not allow me to get the prior position, and this time, I would be prepared and cautious about any of my answers. If we are not learning from our failures, we are not growing. Failure is only failure if you do not learn from it.

The people I would compete against were good candidates. They had no problems speaking English. They had no issues with grammar and had already held director positions at their prior companies. Of the entire group, I was the rookie. If you were looking from the outside, I was the one who was not playing it safe, and everyone thought I would not get it.

Have you ever been in a situation where you were close to achieving something? You were so close it scared you? I was scared to death. I didn't want to lose again. My mentor used to say, "Fear is a lack of confidence. When you can overcome fear, you will succeed." So, if fear is a lack of confidence and the confidence come from practicing, I dedicated myself to practicing all possible questions, the scenarios and most importantly, how I would execute my plan.

Do you remember when you wanted to learn how to drive a car or ride a bike? At first, you were scared to death, but slowly, confidence replaced that fear. Once you were used to the process, you realized it wasn't too difficult. It is the same with everything else in life. We fear approaching someone to ask for help; to try new things; to get into a new social network; to go against our own beliefs, to start a new business, to change your job, your career, all the fear is a lack of confidence. My mentor always said, "The difference between a successful man and an unsuccessful man, is one has no fear while the other one does."

Whatever you are afraid of today, now is the time for you to face it. You only have one life; you only have one chance; you only have today's opportunity to do it. If you believe this is the right thing to do, then go ahead and do it. With these thoughts in mind, I banished my fear. I believed if someone could achieve it, then so could I. It may take me a little longer, but I would do it.

I went to the interview confident I would get the job. I had been preparing myself for this moment for years. My mentor was right. When opportunity and preparation combine, people call it good luck. I was there with the opportunity, prepared to face the new chapter of my life. When the interview ended, I was confident and excited about my performance. I paid attention to my answers and was thoughtful and careful with my responses. I went home happy and told my wife I was sure I would receive a call for the next round.

A couple days later, the call came. I was in the second round. I would interview with the new Vice President of OPS Services. He had been recently hired, and I knew nothing about him. I researched him on LinkedIn and asked some friends more about him. I prepared myself for the interview, but I was also curious about the person I was going up against. I dedicated the next two days to preparing even more, gaining confidence, and planning my new career life. I knew I would get the position this time. I was ready and knew I was the best choice for the job. I had to make sure I conveyed this during the interview.

The day of the interview, I sat fully composed, waiting for my turn. I kept looking to see if I could identify my competitor. I didn't see anyone. While waiting, I saw someone from the office I knew. I asked him who the other candidate was. He said there was no one else. I was the only candidate to make it to the second round. He congratulated me and kept walking. I was so happy. I was here to meet my new boss as well as an interview with him for the position. When it was all over, I got the job.

Church's gave me the opportunity I had worked toward all these years. They believed in me; they trusted me, and most importantly, they respected me as an individual. It was an amazing experience. My growth over the past years was incredible. My new boss is one of the best supervisors I have ever had. He allows me to be me, to show my talents, and to make important decisions for the benefit of the company. I strongly believe Church's Chicken's values embody who I am. We work together to achieve common goals. We always do the right thing, not only for the company but for our people. We want to make sure our team members feel we care about them. We always step up to help others. We do not allow others to fail. We work to leave them better than when they arrived. We also celebrate our differences. We recognize the individuals that makes a difference, who works hard and step up their game.

It took me six years to emerge from depression in Trenton to achieving this level of success. It was far from easy, but I was happy I had accomplished my goal. I am grateful for all the great people I have met and worked with during my time at Church's. I am treated with respect, and I feel valued. I could not ask for a better group to work and achieve my goals with.

There are two questions I am always asked: How did you get into your position? They are surprised because it is not easy for an immigrant, without a college degree, and with English as a second language to get where I have gotten. I give the same answer every time. There are three reasons: I wasn't afraid, I prepared myself for the opportunity, and I mastered my strengths, so others ignored my weaknesses.

Team Building

Developing a champion team has been one of the most valuable contributions to the brand. I worked very hard to develop the people around me, to transform their lives in many ways. I strongly believe confidence is the key to success. When people are confident about their jobs, about themselves and about their abilities, the results are imminent. I understand a powerful and successful leader operates the best when the employees work with a team mentality, each filling a needed role and fulfilling goals.

One of my biggest passions is helping people to discover their strengths and develop to the next level. I love to present an opportunity for the people to grow. I believe in opportunities. I believe everyone should have a chance to demonstrate their talent and ability. What has surprised me over the years is that people do not know themselves or they do not know how to move to another stage of their life or career.

Every year, I've promoted over 60 percent of my team. I spent 90 percent of my time traveling around the USA, spending time with my team, building the most successful team anyone could have. We touched almost every area of the company and supported our people in many ways. One of the things I enjoy most is the transformation of the people once they come to work for me. The lack of confidence, unknown strengths, basic knowledge and they are used to being micromanaged by their prior supervisor. There are many stories I can share with you, but today I want to share Joe's story.

I met him for the first time four years ago. He was a young manager in one of our restaurants in Texas. Church's Chicken has been the only job Joe's ever had. He had never been outside of Texas. He was about 22. On that day, I went to see someone who worked for me, and he was working in Joe's restaurant. Now that I saw Joe, I noticed he was a talented young man. It was impressive how he managed his restaurant; he was sharing with me how many people he has developed in the last few years, and he also asked me what he had to do to be a part of my team. When he asked me these questions, and he shared with me everything he had done, I was seeing someone who believed in what I believed. I left that day happy to see someone so talented.

The time passed, and I didn't see or hear about Joe. Until three years ago, when we were at our annual conference in Houston, Texas. I remembered he was wearing a black suit, the same as me, he shaved his head, the same as me, and he had been following me, trying to get my attention. Finally, he approached me to tell me his goal was to work for me the next year and he was doing everything possible to be on my team. You could tell from his face and the movement of his hands that Joe was nervous. It was not an easy moment for him, but he was willing to achieve his goals and willing to face his fears. He asked me to be his mentor. I think this was fundamental and smart. I knew at that moment Joe would be my next Operations Excellence coach.

A few months later, I asked Joe to fly to Atlanta to meet with me and my boss at the airport. We were sitting in Applebee's, talking with Joe and having lunch when he stopped the conversation to thank me for flying him in. This was his first time flying in an airplane and even getting out of Texas. He was so excited that he felt he had to share this with us. I have been working with Joe for the last two years, and I am proud to say Joe is traveling all over the country. He is confident about his talents and abilities. He is one of our top performers in the company and just to tell you as I am being promoted again to a new role within the cooperation, he is one of the top candidates to take over my current position. Never dream to small, anything is possible if you set your mind to it and ask the right questions. I personally believe he would be a great asset in this role and achieve great things. I wish him the best of luck, just kidding, he is well prepared to meet his destiny.

 Building a great team is not always easy to achieve, you must have a great relationship with others and create a culture of self-development. I constantly do seminars and developmental classes to stay tuned up like a well-oiled machine to better serve my people.

Vulnerability

Showing vulnerability is not always easy. At Church's, I have learned this is a powerful tool and has been one of the major contributors to my success. We are taught that to be vulnerable is to be weak, but it shows how strong a person is when they can be transparent with others. As a leader your ability to be vulnerable translates into buy-in from your followers.

 Now you've been given a glimpse into my journey to success, I ask you to be the author of your own success. Let my failures and setbacks be examples that no matter where you come from or your current situation you can rise to the top when you face your fears. I am no different from you. If I can do it, so can you. In hindsight, my past prepared me for my future, but I had to first embrace the power of discomfort to reach the other side of fear. Right now, I'm living my best life and doing what I love. Always remember that the battle is never over until you quit.

While telling these stories, I've not only had the chance to look back on my life, but to reflect on how my values have changed. When I was younger, I wanted to be rich. Money motivated me, and I wanted a lot of it. Success drove me and I dreamed of living a life full of it. But even though money and success were all I dreamed of at one point, it never completed me. It never filled a void in my heart and soul.

Today, I can care less about being rich. All I want is to is to be a good father, someone who can provide for his children, teach them how to be a good person and marvel at their success along the way. I want to be a good husband—with the ability to be there for my wife during the hardest times and bring a smile to her face and make her laugh daily. Family motivates me. And family completes me.

My journey isn't complete, but today, I'm more interested in my kids' journey. What will they do? Where will life bring them? Have I prepared them enough for their maiden voyage? These are my concerns.

This book's sole purpose was to present my life's struggles and the lessons I've learned from them as a roadmap to success. I only hope that when people finish reading my story, they take their lives into maximum overdrive. Don't feel bad for me or for what I endured. Don't focus on the story; focus on the lessons. Because the feelings I had when these events were happening, have changed.

For example, I've forgiven my mother for her mistakes. I've forgiven my father for his mistakes. Who am I to judge them for their behavior? They gave me the gift of life – a gift impossible to enjoy without screwing up. I have learned to take their mistakes in full stride, to absorb and understand them. I've learned from them, and I try not to make those mistakes with my children. Like everything, these mistakes are now life lessons.

When I was younger, I let my parents' mistakes fester; I didn't address them. As a result, they piled up inside. I didn't become depressed because of my mother or because of my father. I didn't understand how to deal with my internal struggles. I failed to address longstanding issues and did not confront inner demons. I got depressed because my cup overflowed with water.

This shouldn't happen. Don't let things eat away at you. The longer they linger, the more they can hurt you. Throughout my life, I've learned that forgiveness is sometimes the hardest thing to do, but it's also the bravest and strongest thing to do.

In life, the three most important things you can do is forgive, hope and get up when you fail. Forgive those who have wronged you – and don't let the pain they've caused eat away at you.

Hope for the best and reach for the stars. Those dreams of success and family and doing something good are within reach. You have to work hard, but when it all pays off, success will only be sweeter.

Finally, when you fail, and life hits you so hard that you're on the ground, get up. Dust yourself off. And hit back. Hit life with all your might; show it you deserve to be the best you can be. And shine.

Many people fail to manifest their dreams into reality due to the fear of change. The truth is that 20 years from now you will be more disappointed in the things you didn't do than by the ones you did. So go confidently in the direction of your dreams. Don't let fear stop you!

ABOUT THE AUTHOR

Manny Languasco is the Sr. Global Director of Operations of a Global Corporation. He is responsible for over 1,600 restaurants globally. He is a captivating and powerful speaker that has inspired others through his incredible message. Manny comes from very humble beginnings, having been raised in the Dominican Republic. Growing up he had very little, but with the guidance and inspiration of his mentors, he has transformed his life and started the amazing journey to achieving incredible professional and personal success. In 2001, full of dreams for a better life, he took a leap of faith and came to the United States. He was an illegal immigrant, unable to speak English, with only $350 to his name. Within a very short span, he went from homeless and broke, to the CEO of his own multi-million-dollar business.

Learn more at www.mannylanguasco.com